Diary of a D.U.I. Victim

D.U.I. Diary

Anonymous

D.U.I. Crime is 100% Preventable
God Bless the Highway Victims

Order this book online at www.trafford.com
or email orders@trafford.com

Most Trafford titles are also available at major online book retailers.

Scripture quotations marked KJV are from the Holy Bible, King James
Version (Authorized Version). First published in 1611. Quoted from the KJV
Classic Reference Bible, Copyright © 1983 by The Zondervan Corporation.

Print information available on the last page.

ISBN: 978-1-4907-8454-0 (sc)
ISBN: 978-1-4907-8455-7 (e)

Library of Congress Control Number: 2017913724

Trafford rev. 09/29/2017

Trafford
PUBLISHING   www.trafford.com
North America & international
toll-free: 1 888 232 4444 (USA & Canada)
fax: 812 355 4082

Division of Diary

I

Shock and Pain – Sunday, October 20th

Think of the one person you can't live without – gone! Out of your life instantly. The cause, D.U.I. collision by a teen drunk. A teen with a prior "reckless" driving charge. Morning after an all night party, speeding in a Construction Zone, explosive crash: common American Highway tragedy. D.U.I. crime is 100% preventable.

My wife, severely injured in the D.U.I. collision, was a passenger in a car driven by a friend. The drunk teen attempted escape after striking a vehicle in the rear in the fast lane. The drunk driver accelerated and slammed into a second car slamming the car into the stone wall, twice. The car totaled. Two senior citizens escaped death. Modern technology and quick medical response and the grace of God combined to save my wife's life and our friend. The drunk teen and three drunk passengers were unharmed.

A radical change in retirement plans. Surgery and therapy to recover from the physical damage resulting from the D.U.I. collision on October 20th. Medical and Legal turmoil. The pain, a new perception of reality.

Royalty killed in a D.U.I. collision. The homeless run down by drunk drivers. Children slaughtered in crosswalks. Common stories: maimed or murdered victims of D.U.I. carnage. Reaction by the public is sadness for the victim and compassion for the drunk driver. Forgive and return the drunk driver's privilege to operate a motor vehicle. Celebrate with champagne. A brother, neighbor, friend. A husband supporting a son and daughter. Someone caught! Your grandmother?

Recent tragedy, a baby in a stroller run down by a 71 year old female drunk driver. The anguish of the parents is unimaginable.

The rich, middle class, and poor share the American Highway. The middle class, the largest contributor to insurance resources. Least insured the poor; highest coverage to the rich. Do we share the same insurance rules? The highway victims without selection by age, gender, personality. Insurance favors the wealthy and defend the drunk driver. Additional insurance coverage for convicted drunk drivers and statistically dangerous teen drivers and older drivers is not required. Protection for the honest motorist ignored.

$25 million insurance claim paid to recent celebrity family. The passenger, a movie star, killed by the "reckless" driver. Insurance premiums from the poor and middle class motorist pay the bill. D.U.I. motorist premium insurance pays to defend drunk drivers. The insurance system regulates insurance policy. Insurance lobbyist guarantee political acceptance of insurance policy.

Read your policy. Are you protected against D.U.I. tragedy? Did you check the box labeled D.U.I. collision protection? Does your insurance insure the "reckless" teen driver for minimal insurance coverage and defends the insurance policy of driving under the influence of alcohol, speeding in a Construction Zone, attempting to evade capture by authorities? Does your insurance protect the passenger in your automobile?

My wife's story is a story with a common thread – highway pain. Americans disabled each year in traffic collisions exceeds war injury, and sadly more deaths. This story is about surviving. Crash injury, maimed, paralyzed, mental shock. Surviving with injury, with pain. Surviving.

Reading the diary, realize the thoughts appear from our minds stressed by an unordinary situation – a calamity and miracle. The words miracle and luck rarely appear in the diary. Why? Words conditional to God. D.U.I. motorists are guided by the devil.

The thoughts and images detail life after the D.U.I. collision – retirement radically altered. Our thoughts, reflections, tears. A record of conversations; my wife's struggle to regain health, happiness. The work of individuals supporting the recovery process. A timeline of recovery. Like a journalist detailing a story. The fire burning fiercely, daily devouring new acreage. News sources report the fierce D.U.I. car crashes, but seldom the victim hardship after the collision. And penalties for drunk driving is often confidential.

Inserted in the diary, are letters to our lawyer. Additional legal documents complete the information surrounding the D.U.I. collision on October 20th and the future consequences.

A copy of Marsy's Law is printed. Perceptive management is the practice of the insurance agencies. The preconceived, consciously orchestrated data to present as evidence of reality experienced by D.U.I. collision, the distorted truth. A one-sided view to protect the insurance credibility. The diary is spontaneous dialogue and thought. The data factual. Conclusions obviously consistent with fact.

D.U.I. information is recorded on the Police Arrest Report and Criminal Court Judgement Document. Medical Records are not presented – privacy rights. The first day, crash, emergency treatment is described. The hospital care, preparation for surgery. The surgery, hospital care. The nursing home, first day. Days of shock. Robotic attitude. Prayer. Wake-up to a new reality.

Diary excerpt… Day one Sunday Morning, October 20th
UCI Medical Center – Emergency. Directions from my daughter. Race down the highway, stop at the gate, search for close-up parking. None!

Second revolution past Emergency Entrance, brake to avoid pedestrian. Exit to garage, parking space on top level, race to Emergency Room. My wife, bruised face, torso, legs. Hooked to machines to monitor and help her fight for life. A smile, sorry to be less than beautiful. Complete incapacitation.

Two days later, the first surgery – arm repair. Next stop the nursing home.

Every day of our life we witness stupidity, greed, unnecessary suffering. We try to endure misfortune and acknowledge life's mystery. We are grateful for the grace of God.

*********** ********* ********* *********

II

Crash Site

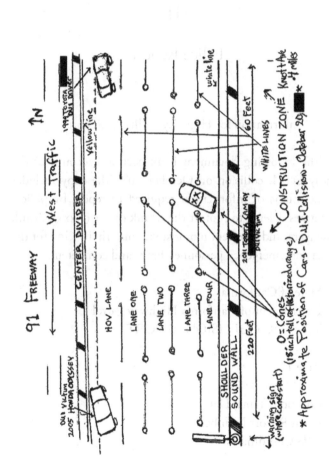

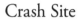

III

Police Report

*** Information for Highway Collision Report

The following document is an accurate account of the deadly D.U.I. collision on October 20th. The copy includes the notations of information required to report by police. All names deleted to protect the drunk driver (Xxxx), drunk passengers, and innocent motorist victims. Thank God for the police and emergency personnel, brave and competent.

State of California
Department of California Highway Patrol
TRAFFIC COLLISION REPORT

Page 1

Location, Time, Date.
Local Report Number
GPS Coordinates

Individuals Involved in Collision
Names, Address, Phone
Physical Description – Sex, Hair, Eyes, Height, Weight
Automobile Identification, License Number
Insurance Carrier

Page 2

Traffic Collision Coding

Property Damage

Seating Position
Safety Equipment
Air Bag
Inattention Codes

Primary Collision Factor
Weather Condition
Lighting
Roadway Surface
Roadway Conditions
Traffic Control Devices
Type of Collision
Motor Vehicle Involved
Pedestrian Actions
Special Information
Other Associated Factors
Movement Preceding Collision
Sobriety, Drugs, Physical

Sketch of Collision – See Collision Diagram

Page 3+

Injured/Witness/Passengers

Name of Injured – Address
Extent of Injury
Description of Injury
Transportation of Injured

Officer Identified

Page 4+

Factual Diagram

Date of Collision, Time, NCIC Number
Officer Identification

Vehicle Points of Rest
Wheel, Reference Point #1, Reference Point #2

Physical Evidence
Description

Location of Physical Evidence
Measurement, Reference Point #1, Reference Point #2

Description of Highway – Lanes, Lines, Barriers,
Measurements, Obstacles
Position of Vehicles

Page 5

Narrative/Supplemental

Date of Incident/occurrence
Time
NCIC Number
Officer ID
Collision Report/Other
Type Supplemental: BA update, Hazardous material, Fatal, School Bus, Hit & Run
City/County/Judicial District
State Highway Related – yes/no

*** Report of D.U.I. Collision – October 20th

Facts – Notification:

I received a call of this collision at 0451 hours. I responded from Beverly Manor south of I-405 and arrived on scene at 0502 hours. All roadway markings appeared to be in good condition upon my arrival. At the time of the collision the roadway had been reduced, to the HOV lane and #1 lane, with 18" reflectorized orange cones. The roadway had been reduced due to ongoing construction. All times, speeds and measurements are approximate. All measurements were obtained by pace.

Scene:

SR-91 at this location is an east west oriented, concrete paved roadway located in the City of Buena Park. There are four lanes for normal traffic and one High Occupancy

Vehicle (HOV) lane for carpool traffic. There is also one lane for traffic exiting the freeway at Beach Blvd. The normal lanes are separated by painted broken white lines. The HOV lane is separated from the normal lanes by painted broken white lines. The north roadway edge is bordered by a solid painted yellow line. The south roadway edge is bordered by a solid painted white line, a ten foot asphalt shoulder and a concrete block sound-wall. East and westbound traffic is separated by a concrete barrier wall. All roadway markings appeared to be in good condition upon my arrival. This collision was contained entirely on the eastbound side of the freeway. This collision occurred during the hours of darkness. Eastbound traffic had been reduced to the HOV lane and #1 lane. All other lanes had been closed off with 18" tall reflectorized orange cones. Approaching the scene there were orange and black advisory signs advising drivers that the right lanes were closed ahead. In addition, there were arrow board signs indicating driver's to merge left and sign boards advising drivers to merge left.

Parties:

Party #1 (Name-Xxxx) was contacted at the scene by CHP Officer A. Axxxx, ID#00000. He was identified by his California Driver's License Identification card and determined to be the driver of the vehicle at the time of the collision by his statement. Passenger One (three in car) confirmation statement and the fact he is the registered owner of V-1.

Vehicle #1 (Black Impala) was located on its wheels in the HOV lane facing e/b. V-1 sustained major front end damage as a result of the collision. P-1 stated that his vehicle had been allowing smoke inside the passenger compartment in the last week. He stated that immediately prior to the collision the passenger compartment filled with smoke reducing his visibility to approximately 60 feet.

Party #2 (Name) was contacted by 2nd Officer B. Bxxxx, ID #00001, at West Anaheim Medical Center. He was identified by his California Driver's License and determined to be the driver of Vehicle #2 by his statement and the fact he is the registered owner V-2.

Vehicle #2 (Honda) was located on its wheels facing east within the construction closure. V-2 sustained moderate damage to the rear bumper, right quarter panel and rear window as a result of the collision. No mechanical defects were noted or claimed.

Party #3 (Name) was contacted at the scene in the back of Care Ambulance #242. She was identified by her California Driver's license and determined to be the driver of the vehicle at the time of the collision by her statement and my observation of her seated in the driver's seat of Vehicle #3.

Vehicle #3 (Toyota Camry) was located on its wheels facing north east in the #4 lane. V-3 sustained major damage to the front, hood, both fenders and both quarter panels as a result of the collision. No mechanical defects were noted or claimed.

Statements:

Party #1 (Name-Xxxx) was contacted at the scene and related in essence the following. (Name) was driving V-1 e/b in the HOV lane at 70-75 mph. (Name) said the passenger compartment began gradually filling with smoke then more quickly. The cabin filled to the point that it reduced his visibility to a distance that he estimated was approximately 60 feet. He stated he recalled seeing red lights then said the vehicles airbags deployed. He said he was unsure if he hit someone or if someone hit him. (Name) said in the last week he began experiencing the cabin filling with smoke when he drove. (Name) was unaware of which vehicle he had collided with.

Party #2 (Name) was contacted at the hospital by 2nd officer and related in essence that he was the driver of V-2 driving e/b in the HOV lane at 60-65 mph when he was hit from behind by an unknown vehicle. This impact pushed his vehicle into the center divider area where it scraped along the center divider wall. He then moved inside the closed off area. Party #2 (Name) related that he was aware of the construction closure and stated that the HOV, #1 and #2 lanes were open but that the other lanes were closed. Party #2 (Name) did not know where Vehicle #3 was in relation to his vehicle prior to the collision or after the impact.

Party #3 (Name) was contacted at the scene by a third Officer Cxxxx, ID#00000, and related in essence the following. She was the driver of Vehicle #3 driving e/b in the #1 lane at 55-60 mph. She stated that traffic was slowing when an unidentified vehicle came up on her left side and collided with her. This sent her out of control across the lanes.

Passenger #1 Impala (Name) was contacted but offered no additional details regarding the collision.

Passenger #2 Honda (Name) was contacted in the back of Care Ambulance but offered no further details regarding the collision.

Passenger #3 Impala (Name) was contacted via telephone and stated that Xxxx was the driver of V-1 at the time of the collision. He stated that Xxxx had been the driver all night. (Name) said they had been in Los Angeles at his friend John and Jane's house. Jane is also known as "Cookie". They arrived at the party about 10 pm and left sometime around 3 am to go to Denny's. (Name) said Denny's was only about 2 miles from the house where they had been. (Name) said they left Denny's sometime past 4:30 am. (Name) stated that he was asleep at the time of the collision. He felt several bumps but did not become alert until after the collision. He stated Xxxx apologized, to (Name) and the other passenger's in Xxxx's vehicle, for having been involved in a collision. (Name) said the other passenger's in Xxxx's car were asleep at the time of the collision as well. (Name) related that after the collision Xxxx explained that he could not see because of smoke reducing his visibility.

Passenger #4 Impala (Name) did not provide a statement. I (police) left a message for passenger #4 but did not receive a return phone call.

Passenger #5 Impala (Name) did not provide a statement. I (police) left a voice mail message for passenger #5 but did not receive a return phone call.

Additional information:

P-1's statement that smoke filled the passenger cabin of his vehicle could not be corroborated by physical evidence or an independent witness. I (Officer) inspected the cabin of V-1 and was unable to locate any evidence to corroborate P.1's claim.

Opinions and Conclusions – Summary:

P-1 was the driver of V-1, driving under the influence of alcohol, traveling e/b on SR-91 in the HOV lane at a stated 70-75 mph, within an established construction closure e/of Knott Ave. directly ahead of V-1. P-3 was the driver of V-3 traveling e/b on SR-91 in the #1 lane at a stated speed of 55-60 mph e/of Knott Ave. ahead and to the right of V-2. Due to P-1's level of impairment, P-1 was driving at an unsafe speed for the conditions. P-1 attempted to avoid colliding with V-2 at the last moment by swerving to the right. The front license plate of V-1 collided with the right rear corner bumper of V-2. This impact pushed V-2 toward the center divider. Due to V-1's excessive speed V-1 continued e/b into the #1 lane overtaking V-3 on the passenger side. The right fender of V-1 collided with the left driver's door turning V-3 to the right and propelling V-3 out of control across all lanes. V-1 continued e/b into the center divider area where it collided with the center divider wall. V-1 traveled back into the HOV lane and came to rest on its wheels facing e/b. V-3 spinning clockwise traveled across all lanes and collided with the left front bumper and left fender with the concrete sound-wall. V-3 continued e/b spinning clockwise and struck the sound wall a second time with the left quarter panel. This impact propelled V-3 out into the lanes within the closure. V-3 came to rest on its wheels facing northeast. Summary based on statement and vehicle damage.

Area's of Impact AOI's:

The area's of impact were located as follows:

AOI #1 v. V-2 was located 6 feet south of the north roadway edge of SR-91 and .4 miles east of the east roadway edge of Knott Ave.

AOI #2 V-1 vs. V-3 was located 14 feet south of the north roadway edge of SR-91 and .4 miles +60 feet east of the east roadway edge of Knott Ave.

AOI #3 V-1 vs. Center divider was located two feet from the north roadway edge of SR-91 and .4 miles +260 feet east of the east roadway edge of Knott Ave.

AOI #4 V-3 vs. Sound-wall was located 10 feet south of the south roadway edge of SR-91 and .4 miles +180 feet east of the east roadway edge of Knott Ave.

AOI #5 V-3 vs. Sound-wall was located 10 feet south of the south roadway edge of SR-91 and .4 miles +220 feet east of the east roadway edge of Knott Ave.

Area of impact determined by statement and vehicle damage.

Intoxication:

Party #1 was initially contacted at the scene by Officer A. Axxxx, ID #00000. Officer Axxxx advised the communications center that P-1 displayed objective symptoms on intoxication. I contacted Xxxx (drunk driver) standing on the right shoulder west of Beach Blvd. Xxxx identified himself as the driver of Vehicle #1 at the time of the collision. The keys for V-1 located in the ignition. Xxxx was identified as the driver of V-1 at the time of the collision by his passenger (Name). He was identified by his California Driver's License. I (Officer) immediately detected the odor of an alcoholic beverage emanating from Xxxx's mouth as he spoke to me. I also observed Xxxx's eyes were red and watery and his speech was occasionally slurred. Xxxx told me he was on his way home from Los Angeles where he had been at a friend's house. He told me he had one Bud Light Platinum beer and some drinks of other beers provided by friends. Xxxx said he started drinking at about 11 pm and finished his beer in about 15-20 minutes. Xxxx stated he did not have any alcohol to drink before the party and told me he did not have any alcohol after leaving the party. Xxxx also stated that he did not consume any alcohol after the collision. Xxxx related that he slept 11 hours the previous night. Xxxx said he ate at Denny's about 15-20 minutes away from the party arriving between 3 and 3:30. Xxxx had a copy of the receipt in his wallet indicating payment was made at 4:19 am. Xxxx said they were coming directly from Denny's before the collision. Xxxx related he did not feel the effects of the alcohol. I explained and demonstrated a series of field sobriety tests which Xxxx was unable to complete as explained and demonstrated. Xxxx was arrested for a violation of CVC section 23153(a) VC per CVC section 40300.5 in or about a vehicle. I (Officer) advised Xxxx of implied consent per CVC section 23612. Xxxx chose a breath test. I transported Xxxx to the Westminster Area CHP office for completion of the chemical test. I setup the AlcoSensor IV-XL evidential breath test and administered Xxxx's requested test. Xxxx was transported to Orange County Jail where he was booked into the custody of the Orange County Sheriff's Department without incident.

Cause:

The cause of this collision was P-1's violation of CVC section 23152(a) driving under the influence of alcohol. An associated factor in this collision is P-1's violation of CVC22350 Unsafe speed for the existing conditions.

Recommendations:

I (Officer) recommend that a copy of this report be forwarded to the North Justice Center District's Attorney's office for the following charges:

2315(a) VC Driving under the influence of alcohol and or drugs causing injury.

The charges can be proven against Xxxx (drunk driver) by the statements obtained from the subject, the statements of parties, the damage to the vehicle, the results of the breath test and the injuries to the parties involved.

Additional Information:

Officer A. Axxxx, ID #00000, is the area PAS coordinator. Officer B. Bxxxx, ID #00001, completed the vehicle report (CHP 180) for V-2 and contacted P-2 and Passenger (Name). Officer A, Axxxx, #00000, contacted P-1 and the passengers in V-1. Officer B. Bxxxx, #00002, completed the vehicle report (CHP 180) for V-2 and contacted P-2 and the passenger in V-2.

Preparer's Name and ID Number

Date

Reviewer's Name

Date

End D.U.I. Report

*********** ********** ********** **********

IV

First Letter to Our Lawyer

Re: Collision of October 20th

Dear Lawyer:

Documents of consent sent to your law office, signed. Thank you for accepting counsel for my wife.

You explained in phone conference the limited insurance coverage of the three insurance agencies representing motorists and passengers involved in D.U.I. collision on October 20th, Sunday morning. Also, explained was the insurance decision for subtraction of insurance money from Civil Trial decision of a settlement for passenger injury by the drunk driver. At present, the Criminal Trial will decide the manner of justice administered for a drunk driving collision in a Construction Zone nearly killing eight humans. The decision for Civil Justice will be determined after the Criminal Trial.

Thank you for explaining Progress Insurance terms that the teen drunk driver's insurance coverage was $25,000 per person with a maximum coverage for all persons not to exceed $50,000. Progress states that there were four injured people involved in the incident. Progress is going to offer its policy to the four individuals that were injured and allow them to reach agreement on how it should be divided. That is, if we should chose not to sue the drunk driver.

We understand our friend, Ms. (Name), insured coverage is $25,000 per person with a maximum for all persons not to exceed $50,000. It may or may not be applicable to the case of my wife.

After examining the Multi-State Insurance of my wife's friend I sent a letter to Multi-State requesting additional information about their D.U.I. Policy or Mission Statement. The complete lack of D.U.I. reference in insurance policy is disturbing. Special reference to racing and weather, nothing about the common highway tragedy – D.U.I. Multi-State refused our request for information.

Following your legal advice, we are documenting the condition of my wife and our change of retirement lifestyle. Diary key words – pain and pill and patience. Learning to move her arm. People at the nursing home are kind; her family and friends help keep her spirit high. This week is currently scheduled for treatment. Wearing leg brace to prevent knee bending. Arm remains immobile – guided therapy movement. My wife cried tears of joy today when her therapist guided her in her wheelchair outside along the sidewalk of the nursing home. First time outside since the collision. Roses lined the walkway.

The scar marks her arm where her flesh is adhering to a titanium plate. X-ray show extent of surgery. The X-ray shocked my sense of proportion. My mind did not visualize the size of the titanium plate – eight screws.

She is walking, baby-steps, still incapable of rising off the ground unaided – no sun tanning on the beach. I fear the pain will continue during our twilight years. Sad. Senseless. The d.d. will never realize how much he hurt someone loved by so many.

Diary entry…
A freeway bump-and-grind, spin-out fender bender? The real picture is a battle scene, twisted metal, mashed flesh. This week's D.U.I. death count, three dead in a morning-after party crash, young deaths. Frightening! Flowers along the curb, familiar sight."

Eight people nearly killed. Mental trauma. My wife damaged, lifeline altered. Pain! Unwanted pain, day and night no end in sight. Tense laughter. Dependent on pain medication. Reflections in the diary add sad tones to the bright light of her survival. She is alive, healing. She is a success story. D.U.I. collisions hurt so many people so badly. Future cars with camera and computer control will end the generations of tragedy.

Amazing the amount of work and misery generated by the D.U.I. A D.U.I. collision is like a bomb threat, you never know where or when the bomb will explode. Please continue the attempt to obtain reasonable restitution from D.U.I. criminal and insurance representatives. Insurance agents need to review Marsy's Law for victim fairness and respect. The court organization, Victim's Rights, sent a copy of Marsy's Law to my wife. Reviewing the Rights.

We have a question. Are the three drunk driver's passengers innocent of the crime? They supported the drunk driver. Handed over the keys with knowledge of the drinking.

Worry about future medical complications and medical cost. I will pass on additional information concerning the D.U.I. collision. The d.d. appears in Criminal Court next month.

My dad was interested in a law career, college in the Depression Era was not possible. I enclose his Civil War novel, a B-western – **Rampant River**. A main character is a lawyer. I changed the timeline, added 30,000 words to my dad's novel. Sequel in production; postponed by D.U.I. collision.

We are grateful for your legal help. The D.U.I. crimes disgrace our country. D.U.I. crime is 100% preventable. God Bless the D.U.I. Victims.

Respectfully,

Name of Victim

*********** ********** ********** ***********

V

Diary – Surgery/Nursing Home

DIARY OF A D.U.I. VICTIM

Wife's Name
Wife's Birthday – October 26, 0000
Lawyer's Name

Case Number 371863
D.U.I. Victim – Name
Sunday, October 20th

October 20th, 21st, 22nd

Shock and pain, day one, day two, day three. Prayer and Faith. Gratitude for my wife surviving the D.U.I. collision. And, Valeria unscathed. And, six strangers without injury.

October 23rd – Surgery.

Marilyn, my wife's sister, recommended a lawyer. Keep a Diary our Lawyer advised. Record life after the D.U.I. collision. Post hell trauma. A diary of facts. A diary of pain.

Waiting room!

Shock and Pain: the voice in the mind exhibits a complexity with adaptation instantaneous.

Recovery room!

My wife talks about her friends and sister visiting and the balloons on her wheelchair. Hospital bed necessary at home. Walk and balance rehab can be from home. The arm treatment is undetermined. Leg injury requires surgery; mobility possible with a cane in time. Cast remains on the leg. Her voice a whisper depressed by drugs.

Concentrate on full recovery. She is shocked by arm surgery pain. Day four. Lucky to be alive. Surgery successful. Wearing knee brace and arm sling.

Wheelchair request. Out patient therapy. Nursing home. Keep careful notes. Purchase cold pack for belly pain from rib damage.

Modern car – saved her life.

Modern Medicine – restores her health.

Friends and Family – protect her soul.

Drive home alone. Miss her voice, the radio talking to mask the silence. Four days. Visits added-up to over thirty hours. Ten hours on freeway traffic to and from the hospital. Miss her laughter.

After surgery she requested the penguin toy to squeeze to increase strength in her arm. Mathew, her grandson collects penguins. She needed the penguin toy. Mathew plans to join the army. The soldier fears disabling wounds. Walking in pain, waking to nightmare. Highway victims receive vicious wounds, similar to combat injury or a bomb blast.

The D.U.I. driver, impossible to vanquish from thought. To extinguish the anger. No wasted thought, his family's problem. My thoughts are devoted to my wife's well being. I visualize healing energy soothing her pain, mending the tear. Prayer to give her strength.

A rapper or diva crash makes news. D.U.I. second generation immigrant? A college student? Teen D.U.I. identity unknown. College, gang, sport freak, terrorist? A teen with future unlimited.

My wife, a model of suburban America. Every dollar reduced by credit charge, gives her money to her children, grandchildren, great-grand child. Senior citizen, retired city employee. My wife does not drink. She does not smoke. My wife experienced tip-top health and vitality prior to the D.U.I. collision.

October 24th – Noontime.

Phone call. Her voice, disappointment. "False alarm. No release from hospital today. The arm. The pain. Exercise arm before release. Milk of magnesia to make me poop. Miserable day. Pain. Dry mouth. Don't want to complain. Take it slow. Extra painful day. Can't shake it. Pain. Feel silly, sleeping at noon."

Technology, the smart phone, my wife loves the smart phone. The phone collection of photos captures every detail, from crash to surgery to scar. Scary!

Amazing how swiftly justice decides the criminal's fate. The D.U.I. driver is out of jail – three hours. Money for bail. Home cooking. Baseball finals.

My wife will not be released today. The pain continues tonight, tomorrow… Medical bills are arriving in the mail. Ambulance.

The weakness in her voice on the phone, frightening. God Bless my darling. She has to take pain pills and sleeping pills. Sleep peaceful, my love. Rest peaceful, sweet darling, sweet dreams.

Leave the house, lock the door. Start the car. Stop for gas. Buy chap-stick for my sweetheart. Listen to the mid-day news. Drive to the hospital to watch my sweetheart sleeping, and pray.

October 25th – Nursing Home.

God protect my wife.

She was crying from the pain of the ambulance ride from the hospital to the nursing home. Settled in a three bed room. She fell asleep while holding my hand.

My wife, my darling, my bride, she is my life. My anchor and guide, amour, paramour, model, soulmate. Every morning, her eyes, lips, touch, the voice to begin the new day.

Life can be abrupt. Ben Franklin said, "be not disturbed by accidents avoidable or unavoidable." Defining a D.U.I. as creating an accident is unacceptable. The man operated a machine with an impaired mental state, deliberately induced and recognizable by the intoxicant. No accident. A man lighting the fuse of a bomb.

Nonchalant acceptance, apathy. Age the constant reminder of mortality. The reality of hours instead of days remaining.

The hopelessness of deterioration. Next generation, nanotechnology, consciousness preserved. Unless the soul finds a new escape from the flesh.

The therapist's husband bought a collapsible boat. He fishes by the **Queen Mary**. The therapist is a bright, spirited young lady, talented, compassionate, dedicated. I'm grateful she guides my wife's therapy after arm surgery. Her laughter is medicine, a gift from God.

Judy, my wife's friend recovering from knee injury at the nursing home is visited by a preacher – Wayne. The preacher says a prayer for my wife. God Bless his soul.

Judy said the psychic lady that visits the nursing home told her to visualize hot barbecue coals on her knees radiating energy. She said to be careful, a tear in the aura produces stroke. She said the flesh consists of globular energy vibrating to the pulse of the universe. I was told the psychic lady wonders the hallways, giving healing power and advice to patients willing to listen or comatose. Sounds harmless.

D.U.I. arrest… Free on $50,000 bail. Public defender. Cost to Public? Substantial. Why? Police report – undeniable evidence.

October 26th – Birthday.
Surgery! Recovery! Scary…
Record thoughts. Facts. The daily race to her bedside…
Smiles…
Pain…

Alone… Driving home… Radio noise…

Traffic tragedy – Sig-alert.
Red Impala ran the red light.
Struck a yellow cab.
Cab driver killed.
Impala driver arrested for D.U.I.

D.U.I. arrest… Free on $100,000 bail. Public defender. Cost to Public? Substantial. Justice?

Strange, the traffic never registered on my mind before collision.

Never repeat radio sig-alert to my wife.

October 26th – Night Visit.

"Shoulder pain will not stop. Staples out yesterday. Pain in my stomach, pain all night long. The shots in the stomach for blood thinning. Ice pack helps.

Visitors. Ruth, Marilyn. Little Ryner riding on the wheel chair. I love you, dear. Ruth joked, *I'll rent the middle bed and spend the night.* Tomorrows activities sound like fun – therapy, tests, pills and shots. Ha! Ha!

Minnesota kids called. Pearl talked for an hour. Wayne, preacher gave a prayer. Under the circumstances a good birthday.

Marilyn gave me a cupcake, chocolate with a swirl of frosting. Calls from Marilyn's boys. Plant from Tom and family. Your sisters cards, perfect.

The casino lady gave Valeria her points.

Nice pleasant birthday, everyone has been kind.

Cards. Three balloons. Cupcakes.

And the best gift. You, sweetheart."

I leaned over the bed and kissed my sweetheart.

Note – Buy Bottle Holder, water, freeze two bottles, buy ice packs, ice block. Medical advisor called from Utah, questionnaire from Quality Insight, medical survey group. I could not talk about my wife. I could not talk about the nursing home. My mind went blank. Too close to the collision. My thoughts are influenced by emotional stress. Too early to ask questions of such a sensitive nature. Incredible the business of people watching people watching people, people, people.

Note: Information on insurance for lawyer. My wife's friend's car insurance coverage for passenger is minimal. Drunk teen driver insurance is minimal. Pictures of black and blue face and torso. X-Ray of titanium plate in arm. Notebook for Faith. Hardware store – eye glass with light.

October 27th – Morning Visit.

"Good Morning sweetheart."

"Just finish breakfast, toast, egg, cereal, cranberry juice.

Sleep pill leaves me lethargic, awake before midnight, before four. T.V. on too loud, turned down. Anyway, going to be a beautiful day. I take shower today. Braces off. Haven't been clean for a couple days."

She jokes about wearing a diaper like her great-grand daughter, Madalyn Rose. They both are learning to walk. Life is precious. Fragile and frivolous.

October 27th – Therapy Session.

"In the therapy room we bounced a balloon back and forth. We bounce a balloon to exercise my right arm, coordinate my balance. When will the left arm come back into play? Patience, slow progress is best.

Dumbbells next. To stretch and flex the uninjured arm.

Newest medicine… Hydromorphone (Dilaudid) to numb pain.

Step forward. Step back. Repeat – twenty times. Patience therapist exercise the injury. Lift the leg, repeat twenty times. Side to side. Cha, cha, cha. Up to the toes, rock the feet, heel-toe, heel-toe. Rock & Roll.

Now a daredevil climb up the steps. Good leg up, bad leg down. The therapist, Jessell, holds my belt, laughs and encourages."

October 28th

Copy lawyer papers tomorrow, copy pictures – car – emergency room – surgery. Organizing papers is an excellent skill. Page #99. Imagine the papers to send the d.d. to jail. The insurance papers, medical, legal – thousands of papers.

No medical complication for the uninjured d.d. and three drunk passengers. Lawyers control the d.d's fate. Life returns to a normal routine – party time?

No guarantee for longevity or health. A brain aneurism kills indiscriminately, hidden in unsuspecting subjects. Auto collision is random selection. Alcohol and driving is suicidal denial, zero respect of life. Alcohol represses the adrenal energy to activate alert reaction. Alcohol impairs awareness of existing conditions.

The activation of auto control in future autos will end generations of suffering where human control is distorted or distracted. Today, jet aircraft land by remote control. Cameras see everything, panorama view. Computers guide the plane to a safe landing, every time. Robotic cars with cameras and computer analysis will guide the future car. The camera will always see a red light and stop the car.

October 29th

Understanding what was lost. Understanding the pain. Attempting forgiveness, failing. Understanding, the d.d. survives and thrives.

Life is precious and fragile.
Life is a profound.
Life is a passionate gift.

"For his anger endureth but a moment:
In his favor is life:
Weeping may endure for a night,
But joy cometh in the morning."

Psalm 30

October 30th

Appointment for dental – 8:00 a.m. My wife's precise scroll, the reminder on the calendar date. Linda, the receptionist, answered the phone.

Reschedule dental appointment for my darling. Wife recovering from a D.U.I. collision. Misery and anger flaunted my voice tone.

A pause. Her sincere sympathy. She said her mother was killed by a drunk teen foreign exchange student. He fled the country. Her mother was fifty-four.

So many years denied her mother.

God Bless her family.

College, institutes of higher learning. Solving problems, discovery. Football and academic perfection. And frat parties, tailgate parties, holiday parties, graduation parties. Eighteen, nineteen, twenty – college students analyzing alcohol by personal experience.

College statistic for drunk driving? College effort to prevent drunk driving? College drunk driving deaths? Mission statement!

October 31st

The greatest theft is not gold or jewels. The greatest theft is time. Steal the hour of a life. An hour to romance, laugh, cry. Our time! Steal Halloween with family and friends.

My wife gives her time to her family and friends. She helped plan and execute her high school reunion. Last year she was a crutch to her friend Ruth, undergoing Chemo Therapy. Her credit cards exhibit her generosity to Daneil, Mathew, Cathy, Nick, Rayette, Misty – her grandchildren. Baby great-grand daughter, Madalyn Rose does not grasp the significance of the credit card, yet. Great grandma will teach her.

My wife is a very active woman. She travels on bus tours with the retirement organization. I tag along – Fillmore Train Ride, Julian Gold Mine, Space Shuttle Museum, Reagan Library, Puppet Studio, **Iowa**, L.A. Times. (The L.A. Times refused to publish my article about Bell High School students, 50 million words on the corrupt mayor, no, can't print 600 words from the students). Dodgers and Angels stadiums.

With her sidekick, Valeria, she helps support the Indian gambling casino. She held her granddaughter's wedding in our backyard. Time. Time. Time. Time. Time. Her time is well spent. Decorating the house front with Halloween animation. A pumpkin boy, witch and Casper ghost. The skeleton hangs in the window. Not this year!

Currently, her time is consumed by rehab exercise. One hour equals three days.

What justice does the thief receive? Perhaps the time of any individual is inconsequential. We sleep half our lives. No great loss? D.U.I. detention, three hours in jail. Piece of cake. Play poker with a cellmate.

Happy Halloween!

November 1st

The day is already planned and spent. Unlike retirement freedom of time. Copy documents for lawyer. Pictures, insurance forms, medical correspondence. Print a picture of Madalyn Rose for my darling patient to hang by her bedside. Her roommate Joey is going home. Faith has a chance to move to the bed by the window. However her right arm would be against the wall. Draft? Bright light? Street noise? Decisions...

Under normal conditions, I would be completing my second book of poetry. I've had some success with my poetry – Writer's Digest Honorable Mention in 2011. I recently read – **Sugarloaf Mountain Trails**. High Sierra poems.

Faith gives my poems to people at the nursing home. She's editing expert, proofreader, spell check. Promotional analysis and number one fan.

As a writer I earn $350 per hour. Future income is considered the primary source of receiving the salary generated. Total royalty to date is low, low, low. However, my venture into the eBook publishing designates me as a pioneer in the new eBook industry. I'm proud of that fact. Promotion, marketing is 75% of the writing business. Writing is a challenge, promotion a chore.

My wife is my muse. She inspires, congratulates, encourages...

November 2nd – Thank God for cell phones.

Phone Call...

Ring-ring.

Pick-up message. "This is Faith. At the tone please record your message. Have a wonderful day."

"Honey, I miss you. I'll call in a moment."

The fear of loss, wow. The empty line. Senseless worry. She is listening to her tape. Ring-ring-ring.

"Hello."

"May I speak to the man of the house?"

"Sorry, wrong number."

"Sorry."

Hang-up.

Wrong number. A hasty hang-up. What if? A girl's voice. A nurse. Who?

Phone message of joy. Message of doom.

Third ring-ring, ring-ring.

"Talking to Rayette. Tom and Nick are in the forest deer hunting."

Her first husband, Steve, isn't hunting this year.

"Green beans, chicken, mashed potato for dinner. Applesauce. Love you, honey.

Pain killer not delivered by pharmacy.

O.K. not bellyaching. I shall see you later."

Note: Pack in car: Water. Banana. Two coat hangers. Robe.

Time: Drive to nursing home – 47 minutes. Traffic cones, one lane closed.

November 3rd – Night, alone.

Can you imagine your son or daughter, college student or new employee, driving drunk after a late, late night party, racing on the Freeway, 75 m.p.h. in a Construction Zone, rear ending a couple in a sedan, speeding across lanes and smashing into a car carrying two older women driving 55 m.p.h. Can you imagine your teenager facing the policeman, explaining smoke in the car obscuring vision, failing the breath test for alcohol? The three male passengers (ages 18-22) did not see what happened, asleep during impact #1 and impact #2.

My wife is a light sleeper. She sometimes watches a midnight movie dated to nostalgic past. The family plots, soapy dramas, thrillers. Now, she fights pain all night, drugged by pain medicine and sleep pills.

Phone call... "Misty has a robe to drop off on the table on the back porch. I need the robe. Bring the robe to me tomorrow.

I'm slipping and slouching in bed. My body looking for a normal position. Then, maybe I can sleep. Headache at dinner. Looking forward to sleeping pill.

The psychic lady stopped by. She said when the body is critically injured, the aura ripped open, the soul will escape the body. Impossible for a soul to leave a healthy body, or damaged body. Especially when the soul is comfortable. Displacing the soul by unnecessary violence, a serious offense. The way of fate is a mystery.

She visits every week, a least once, sometimes more. She lives near-by. She's harmless. Tells fortunes, gives psychic cures, talks to Spirits. She said my mother is painting in heaven.

I love you darling. Love you, love you, love you."

November 4th

Amazing how the mind extracts information connected to a particular subject – collision. Killed eight, injured thirty. Bus crash on Highway 38, near the Ranger Station, San Gorgonio Wilderness. Avoidable, ignored safety problems, tour bus. We forget swiftly, the day's tragic events on roads we drive along everyday. The crash caused by neglect. Flowers along the highway, the cluster of crosses, the end.

November 5th – Silence is Golden.

Can't seem to catch-up on tasks – mail, visit to nursing home, pick-up medicine, pay bills, get gas, visit the nursing home – eat! First order of importance, review Victim's Rights document – Marsy's Law. Send letter to lawyer; insurance information and questions. Our legal confusion about victim rights and criminal rights.

Turning a corner on the way to visit my wife a driver in a pick-up truck illegally cut in front of my car. I beeped. The driver followed me, cursing. What has happened to courtesy on the road? Self-control! I learned a lesson today, don't beep when a road mistake happens. Safer! Road Rage can be set off by a gesture.

********** ********** ********** **********

VI

Second Letter to Our Lawyer

Dear Lawyer:

Salutations! Happy days, peaceful nights. "We choose to do things not because they are easy, but because they are hard." JFK

Searching for D.U.I. information Letters sent to insurance and probation and Victim's Rights reveal interesting facts. Cooperation limited, representatives of convicted D.U.I. will not provide Progress Insurance policy. Progress will not provide Colossus Scale. D.U.I. current criminal status unknown, Probation silent. Criminal trial postponed, new date February 10th. No explanation. Possibly, Civil Trial will allow access to D.U.I. insurance and license information.

Enclosed is Criminal Trial Restitution Form sent by Probation Department. I'm confused on the procedure for collecting D.U.I. information and Reasonable Restitution. Request for information from Probation Officer returned without response. New Probation Officer assigned.

Exceptional number of workers engaged by D.U.I. criminal activity.

Our naive assumption concerning "high risk" insurance necessary for "reckless" teen drivers is incorrect. Foolish assumption, that "reckless" or convicted "D.U.I." motorists require "high risk" insurance. The insurance premium increases, not the coverage. And, the report of a D.U.I. collision to insurance agencies from a passenger victim is optional, encouraging fraud and deception. Probation Court will not provide driving record or insurance policy of D.U.I. motorist.

In a letter to my wife the insurance settlement "Colossus Scale" proposed by Progress Insurance is still a mystery. Your original insurance information is understandable. Insurance money for injured passengers is limited. Minimum restitution by Progress defending the convicted D.U.I. motorist policy sold to a teen with a "reckless" driving charge, no job, a drinking problem exhibits bad business practice, but legal. Multi-State and Infinite support the Progress business practice – low cost insurance, low cost coverage, "high risk" driver. Very disconcerting to see the interpretation of D.U.I. law regarding insurance and criminal punishment.

Providing low coverage insurance for convicted D.U.I. motorists is wrong. Defending the policy is accepting a breach of the insurance agreement by the drunk motorist. However, policies inspected had no reference to D.U.I criminality. Racing, lightning strike, malicious mischief, flood, etc. Nothing about the common D.U.I. deadly highway danger. Less insurance equals less highway safety, laws allowing dangerous motorist limited insurance is wrong.

The policy of limited insurance for "reckless" and "D.U.I." motorists must be endorsed by all insurance agencies. The collaborated effort of three insurance agencies to minimize restitution for passenger victims is understandable. D.U.I. policies increase insurance money account; injured victims decrease the insurance money account. Victims without insurance are castaways. Assume a child (God forbid) passenger is injured – insurance defends the drunk's policy against a legal alternative. A legal alternative of reasonable restitution proposed by a lawyer paid by the victim. The concession to the intoxicated driver evidently maintains justice, fair play and respect for a misguided teen or confused female like the recent celebrity D.U.I.

In the twisted logic of legal interpretation the drunk motorists becomes an uninsured motorist when his policy is voided for breach of contract rules. Unfortunately, nothing in the insurance policies prevents drunk driving or defines D.U.I. policy. Can a contract be broken illegally without conditions in the contract to provide for the criminal action? Insurance can justify switching coverage for all possible legal situations.

Civil Trial is the next step in our effort to receive Reasonable Restitution for D.U.I. collision on October 20th. Minimal D.U.I. insurance money contested in trial and separate restitution from D.U.I. resources – particularly parent financial support – bail, lawyer, fine, plus restitution.

A Multi-State letter enclosed indicating no support for passenger victim injured in D.U.I. collision. Property damage questionable – wardrobe replacement and dental repair?

Premium collected from D.U.I. criminals is probably spent defending the policy of the drunk motorist. Restitution from premium collected from D.U.I. criminals is absurd. Insurance is not in the business of compensating injured passengers or improving highway safety. Replacing the auto is primary purpose; air bag technology protects the passenger.

The criminal D.U.I. is protected by the legal system. The drunk driver returns to the privilege of driving without increase of insurance coverage to protect the honest motorist. And, the insurance agency collects a premium for funds to protect the rights of the D.U.I. And, business is booming! Thirteen D.U.I. convictions on one recent D.U.I. arrest – "catch and release policy." One thousand D.U.I. arrests on Thanksgiving. Catch and release.

Victim's Rights indicate restitution for victims. Perhaps a request to the insurance company to consider funneling a portion of the criminal funds collected from convicted D.U.I. policies into reasonable restitution on serious bodily injury victims from a D.U.I. collision. The extra money for "high risk" insurance does not cost the insurance agency extra money to send a monthly bill. According to "Victim's Rights" money collected from the convicted criminal belongs to the victims. Victims are entitled to money generated by the convicted criminal. Insurance cost does increase to cover a convicted D.U.I. policy. The extra fee can be defined as a criminal fine. The added fee for "high risk" insurance for convicted drunk drivers should belong to the victims. Marsy's Law #3, Section C: *All monetary payments, monies, and property collected from any person who has been ordered to make restitution shall be first applied to pay the amounts ordered as restitution to the victim.*

Reasonable Restitution for the injured passengers is contested. The senior citizen passenger, nearly killed by four drunks in a D.U.I. collision in a Construction Zone, dismissed by three insurance agencies – victim's lawyer proposal for legal alternative rejected. Three insurance agencies determine the passenger victim is underinsured. The insurance of a car struck by a drunk's car denies victim's injury claim. Convincingly, the law is on the side of the D.U.I. criminal.

Insurance agencies do not need to cooperate in the settlement of an insurance claim. Prosecutors and judges agreed with "catch and release" justice for a drunk driver. Crashing eight humans into near death in a Construction Zone, acceptable level of D.U.I. destruction and injury – no death. A Civil Trial judge defending victim's rights against the D.U.I. insurance lawyer and public defender is a gamble – odds favor the D.U.I.

Helping a D.U.I. victim is commendable. A claim for reasonable restitution from insurance was ethical and legal. No reason justifies the refusal by the insurance agency for reasonable restitution. Defending the D.U.I. minimal restitution is wrong. The insurance agencies ignore the legal proposal of a senior injury passenger in favor of a drunk driver's broken insurance policy. Double amount of minimal settlement to include spouse loss dismissed by insurance agencies.

Like the question of good or evil a decision of conscious universally accepted. Perhaps a Civil Trial judge with victim empathy will order insurance D.U.I. premium funds as settlement restitution for D.U.I. victim. Perhaps double restitution for a Construction Zone collision. Property lose, dental damage. Civil Trial will clarify the insurance position defending a drunk's policy against victim's legal alternative. Please continue the legal procedure and inform us of possible Civil Trial after Criminal Trial verdict on February 10th.

God Bless the Highway Victims.

Respectfully,

Victims of D.U.I.

********** ********** ********** **********

VII

Victim's Rights – Marsy's Law

District Attorney (Name)
County of Orange

Defendant: Xxxx
Court Case Number: 00RF0000
Victim Witness: 000-000-0000

www.orangecountyda.com

This is your notice of Victim Rights in the above case. If you have questions or input in this case, please contact the Victim Witness Program at the telephone number listed above. If you would like to check on hearing dates for this case, go to www.occourts.org and use the defendants name and case number. Please be advised that criminal cases may be resolved as early as the first court appearance. Experiencing loss as a result of criminal activity may be a challenging experience. The District Attorney's Office is working to ensure that justice is done in your case. Thank you for the opportunity to serve you. For additional legal information and victims' resources, please visit www.orangecountyda.com.

Victims' Bill of Rights
Your rights under Marsy's Law include:

1... Fairness and Respect. To be treated with fairness and respect for his or her privacy and dignity, and to be free from intimidation, harassment, and abuse, throughout the criminal or juvenile justice process.

2... Protection from the Defendant. To be reasonably protected from the defendant and persons acting in behalf of the defendant.

3... Victim Safety Considerations in Setting Bail and Release Conditions. To have the safety of the victim and the victim's family considered in fixing the amount of bail and release conditions for the defendant.

4... The Prevention of the Disclosure of Confidential Information. To prevent the disclosure of confidential information or records to the defendant, the defendant's attorney, or any other person acting on behalf of the defendant, which could be used to locate or harass the victim or the victim's family or which disclose confidential communications made in the course of medical or counseling treatment, or which are otherwise privileged or confidential by law.

5... Refusal to be Interviewed by the Defense. To refuse an interview, deposition, or discovery request by the defendant, the defendant's attorney, or any other person acting on behalf of the defendant, and to set reasonable conditions on the conduct of any such interview to which the victim consents.

6... Conference with the Prosecution and Notice of Pretrial Disposition. To reasonable notice of and to reasonably confer with the prosecuting agency, upon request, regarding, the arrest of the defendant if known by the prosecutor, the charges filed, the determination whether to extradite the defendant, and, upon request, to be notified of and informed before any pretrial disposition of the case.

7... Notice of and Presence at Public Proceedings. To reasonable notice of all public proceedings, including delinquency proceedings, upon request, at which the defendant and the prosecutor are entitled to be present and of all parole or other post-conviction release proceedings, and to be present at all such proceedings.

8... Appearance at Court Proceedings and Expression of Views. To be heard, upon request, at any proceeding, including any delinquency proceeding, involving a post-arrest release decision, plea, sentencing, post-conviction release decision, or any proceeding in which a right of the victim is at issue.

9... Speedy Trial and Prompt Conclusion of the Case. To a speedy trial and a prompt and final conclusion of the case and any related post-judgment proceedings.

10... Provision of Information to the Probation Department. To provide information to a probation department official conducting a pre-sentence investigation concerning the impact of the offense on the victim and the victim's family and any sentencing recommendations before the sentencing of the defendant.

11... Receipt of Pre-Sentence Report. To receive, upon request, the pre-sentence report when available to the defendant, except for those portions made confidential by law.

12... Information About Conviction, Sentence, Incarceration, Release, and Escape. To be informed, upon request, of the conviction, sentence, place and time of incarceration, or other disposition of the defendant, the scheduled release date of the defendant, and the release of or the escape by the defendant from custody

13... Restitution.

A. It is the unequivocal intention of the People of the State of California that all Persons who suffer losses as a result of criminal activity shall have the right to seek and secure restitution from the persons convicted of the crimes causing the losses they suffer.

B. Restitution shall be ordered from the convicted wrongdoer in every case, Regardless of the sentence or disposition imposed, in which a crime victim suffers a loss.

C. All monetary payments, monies, and property collected from any person who has been ordered to make restitution shall be first applied to pay the amounts ordered as restitution to the victim.

14... The Prompt Return of Property. To the prompt return of property when no longer needed as evidence.

15... Notice of Parole Procedures and Release on Parole. To be informed of all parole procedures, to participate in the parole process, to provide information to the parole authority to be considered before the parole of the offender, and to be notified, upon request, of the parole or other release of the offender.

16... Safety of the Victim and Public are Factors in Parole Release. To have the safety of the victim, the victim's family, and the general public considered before any parole or other post-judgment release decision is made.

17... Information About These 16 Rights. To be informed of the rights enumerated in paragraphs (1) through (16).

Definition of Victim

A 'victim' defined under the California Constitution as "a person who suffers direct or threatened physical, psychological, or financial harm as a result of the commission or attempted commission of a crime or delinquent act." (Cal. Const., art. 1, 28(e).)

Victim Witness

Your local Victim Witness Assistance Center can provide advocacy and specific information on local resources, the Victim Compensation Program, nonprofit victim's rights groups and support groups. You may also contact the Attorney Generals Victim Services Unit 1-877-433-9069.

********** ********** ********** **********

VIII

Nursing Home Rehab

November 6th – Good-bye Joey.

Mail health form for ambulance cost.

Joey, my wife's roommate, leaves for home today, walking out the door, she passed the t.v. remote control to my wife. They will keep in touch.

Pills have not arrived with lunch. Walking exercising with the pain is impossible.

90 day pill supply, picked up at the pharmacy, the cost was correct. My wife is an efficiency expert in our home. Tough to play the game with half the team missing.

November 7th – Sea Poems.

Read sea poems to my wife. My effort with words is to create an image of beauty. I pray the poems fill my wife's mind with the gentle sound of the surf, the mystic blue of the sky and the play of the dolphins. I pray my poems erase the violence and pain inserted into her mind by the drunk driver.

November 8th – Bar Stop #1.

There is a hammock moon tonight with Venus resting near. A quarter crescent shinning bright, peaceful. The cars zoom past on the boulevard, day shift ended, time for the drink. The lure of relaxation and quiet contemplation. One drink. You can handle one drink. Traffic is light. Short-cut to home.

The sport bar where golf buddies meet. A want-a-be Romeo. Two fisted drinker – always sober. Macho man. Fun. Fun. Fun. A short ride home. One stop-sign. Left turn. Two more blocks. One. Zero. Crunch. The neighbor's cat.

November 9th – Boring Stuff.

Before the d.d. mauled my wife. Crushed and ripped like a lion attack. I was finalizing the pages of a second book of poems and typing pages from a new novel – curiously concerning the life of a young person released from jail. I write an accurate contemporary story – however, the fiction story and writer weave together, impossible to separate. Telling the d.d. story is fact, a narrative with direct connection to all the damn drunks that maim and kill on American highways. The nursing home people are real. My wife is real.

The d.d. is unknown. A teen. A drunk teen. No identity. A highway terrorist?

The lawyer instructed, "Keep a diary, a journal. Record your wife recovering. Record what happens. Treatment, drugs, day-to-day return to health. Day to day pain.

Hot story. The college student, 2nd generation immigrant, ripped from family and jailed, that is a t.v. episode. Gang violence. Misguided youth.

Older women, a nursing home, hardly news worthy.

November 9th – Noon.

Strange, evident guilt challenged. Truth twisted. Refusal to reply. Law interpretation. Man to man, impossible to shake hands. No apology, or well wish. Simply, the static discharge of money to sustain the costs. Compensation to assuage despair. Incarceration awarded the guilty. Time to realize the mistake ruins lives. Interaction between people requires rules. In the nursing home, in the prison. One rule: never make another person's life more difficult.

*****Pill Schedule*****
Note paper of effort to keep track of pill schedule.
3:30 p.m. Pain Pill.
10:26 p.m. medicine… potty twice in diaper.
Sunday: 1:13 a.m. medicine… pain pill.
Sunday: 8:00 a.m. pain pills.
Pills… 12:30 p.m.
Pills… 1:45 p.m.
ZZZZZZZZZ
ZZZZZZZ
ZZZZ
Pills… 5:45 p.m.
Pills… 10:00 p.m. / Monday 8:30 a.m.
Monday 11:00 a.m. pills.
5:30 p.m. pills.
Tuesday 8:45 a.m. pills.

14-A
Renal R
Percocet Q 6 HRS routinely as needed Q 4 HRS

November 10th

A woman, very ill, yelling, crying for help all night was moved out of one room and into my wife's room. New room mate ejected from her original room. Faith won't complain. Faith is a cheerful lady. Faith, my darling Faith. In so much pain. And the prescription medicine waiting for doctor approval. Weekend coming, new arrivals. Soon, darling, soon you will be home.

The d.d. is home. Talking to his friends who saw nothing that terrible morning. Party night. Every story needs a party. College party, keg of beer, sex and drugs. Wild music, fast cars, football, ra-ra. The beat goes on.

Confronting father knows best. Tears, but a stern denial. "I wasn't drunk, dad. I was tired. We stopped for breakfast. The Construction Zone obscured by smoke in the car. I was blinded. The car I hit slowed suddenly. The second car weaved into my lane. Honest dad. I wasn't drunk. This wasn't my fault. The construction signals confused the other drivers. The smoke blinded me. Honest dad."

Honesty, the tradition of America – George Washington's Apple Tree. Individualism – Henry David Thoreau. Football, beer, rock-&-roll. The legacy of generations, the complete American. College degree, fancy car, super-size television, credit cards. Church membership, optional. Unionized voter. And the right to do whatever. Don't get caught – mantra. Someone always there to bail you out, if caught.

You'll be home soon darling. Five more days, maybe. No more diaper change. You can control the t.v. remote. You can water your flowers. No lifting, darling. Not even Madalyn Rose.

Recently, the prison inmates demanded improved medical treatment, the judges agreed. The older folks in the nursing homes never demand, the Gray Wolves work.

The d.d. probably in jail listening to heavy metal on headphones. Jail time to think about the collision – the consequences of criminal behavior.

Correction, drunk driver is out on bail – $50,000.

Note...
Cold Water
Check Book – Bottom drawer by chair. Check book in bag.
Call Dorothy – Avon Lady

November 11th
Our granddaughter, Misty, is a talented tattoo-artist. I suggested a vine with red roses and bluebells to disguise the scar on my wife's arm. The thought of adding pain to the arm with ink needles was insensitive.

I cannot think of injecting humor into conversation with my wife. Avoiding d.d. reference is paramount. I read her my sea poems. We talk about pain. Belly, arm, leg, tailbone, headache. All that pain without reason. Dying isn't a problem. Dying for a stupid reason is a sin. Mother Nature leads the majority to the invisible new home.

I wonder what the Psychic Wanderer knows about the Here-After. Note: ask Faith to ask her when she appears.

Lifetimes, hundreds of years, represented in the faces of the residents of the nursing home. The oldest resident, thirty years. Eleven discharged during my wife's tenure. Three died, peacefully. The age span at the home, 65 to 103. Eighty maximum occupancy. Swift, professional treatment.

The goal – discharge. Make room for a new patient for convalescent care. A revolving door.

My wife suggested I use the word approximately, beside the nursing home statistics. Numbers always lie. The number of nursing homes within a twenty mile radius, thirty. This is all approximate. Our reality shifted the day of the D.U.I. collision. Ignore that fact, darling. I love you; that is what you need to hear. The skipped repeat of a broken record – I love you.

My wife will be pleased by these hundreds of words expressing my deepest love and devotion and attention. I love you. I love you. I love you…

Ruth is visiting. She received Chemo-therapy last year. Her son lives by the Trinity River in Northern California with his wife and two teen girls. Ruth is a rock. Thank God for true friends.

November 12th – Night phone talk.

"I miss you – write that down in our journal. I miss you. In the medicine cabinet, eye drops. Not the red-out. Eyes hurting. Headache monumental. Exercising, a mile walking to the restroom. I love you."

Any distraction from pain is a plus. Few words, pain, sleep dearest.

"I love you."

District attorney, police officer, jailor, bondsman, lawyer, ambulance drivers, insurance agents, hospital receptionist, nurses, surgeon, therapist. D.U.I. takes away the people needed to help in natural emergencies. Fire, falls, children injury. D.U.I. needless waste of valuable resources. **The**

Magnificent Obsession – one heart machine – two patients. Rock Hudson stared in the movie.

November 13th

I look at my chair on the back patio where I read books. Spider webs tangle the legs. Dust covers the cushion. Scientists are creating spider strength wire, I read that fact in a magazine in the hospital surgery waiting room.

Today I bought a seat cushion for my wife. Tailbone pain. My step-dad suffered lower back pain. In high school a jokester pulled his chair away and Russel fell on his tailbone. Age and arthritis equal severe pain. He served our country in the Marines.

Bought a second cushion for my wife's friend, Judy, at the nursing home. Any way to increase comfort: ice pack, cushion, word puzzle book, books on tape, the newspaper funnies, lemon drops, iced water, pictures and cards. Whatever is needed to comfort. Balloons!

Pills and exercise. Pills and exercise. Breakfast, lunch and dinner. Bingo in the afternoon. Pills and sleep. The routine continues. Soon she will be home, next week perhaps.

At home the exercise will continue and the pills. Of course the pain.

It cannot happen to the one you love. What are the odds? Statistically, everyone in America will be robbed once and in one auto accident. In Southern California one third of the women are raped. It cannot happen to the one you love. God will protect her soul.

Cobwebs on the back of the chair. Busy spiders. Busy people. Busy freeway. Everyone has an agenda to follow. I read in the afternoon. Soon, I'll return to my mundane pattern. And watch my wife water flowers – orchids, poinsettias, roses, tulips, daffodils…

We'll take a walk on the pier. I'll finish my sea poems. We'll hang Christmas lights. Back to normal. A little older. No wiser. Spinning our own web.

Reckless endangerment of eight lives. The bus crash killed eight on Highway 38. A sunny Wednesday morning. Six, eight, twelve deaths, sensitivity to life? Empathy! The callous acceptance. A car crash casualty. Excellent television coverage. What can you do?

Slow down, follow the highway rules. Stay alert! Simple, don't be a fool.

November 14th – Phone Call at 7:00 a.m.

"12-6-12-6 schedule."

My wife talks, disorientated.

"Pain pills arrived. Ate whole dinner. Cooked vegetables, mushrooms and ravioli and garlic bread. Good! Cinnamon baked apples. Delicious meal.

Pain pills arrived. Eight, then start again at midnight. Save newspapers. **Dirty Dancing** now on Family Channel 28. Missing you. Slot machine game in the recreation room. Tired. Love you."

"Sweet dreams, honey."

"Love you."

My wife tapes the television shows. Soap and drama. Fast forward the commercials. I'm watching reruns and commercials.

Note: refill dish-soap bottle. Water flowers. Gas! Wash the bed sheets. Shower. Buy bananas for my dearest. Print new picture of Madalyn Rose. Flip the knife sharpener blades.

The average human mind remembers seven things. I have the coat hangers, ice packs, cushion. Freeze the water bottles. Ambulance bill – two. Match bill with medical coverage – mail. Dinner – another sandwich. The complexity of our minds, instantaneous images, detail recalled.

The smell of her perfume scents the hallway. She is a Scorpio. Sex is a frequent happening. Kisses morning to night. I'm a Gemini, I miss her doubly badly.

November 15th – Wake-up pain.

I think I'm experiencing sympathy pain. Leg pain, back pain, arm pain. Tears, release pain.

Parents cry for a fool. And money determines fate. Think positive!

Soon my wife will be home. Her pink robe whirls in the dry cycle. She needs coat hangers and her slippers. A siren in the distance, toward the nursing home. A busy route, a dangerous drive.

November 15th – Afternoon Phone Call.

Ring-ring. No response.

Problem, conflict, setbacks, crisis and solution. The novel on the back shelf.

At the tone please record: "Hi babe, called to check on your condition. I love you."

Repeat call in twenty minutes. Ring, ring again… I hit the wrong button. I hit the same button – ignore.

Correctly dial, leave a message at the tone. "Hi love. Watching football. Player, 280 pounds, carried off with a bungled knee. How was the movie **Dirty-Dancing**. I'll be there soon dear."

Thirty minutes goes past, fast. Next call. Connection.

We talk about the medicine.

"I can't understand the problem. Medicine, not given. Anyway, dinner coming soon."

"I miss you, honey. I'm writing in the journal. Problem, now is the typing. I'll print out the injury pictures for the lawyer. Be brave."

"I love you."

"Bye angel."

I hang up the phone, exit the house, enter the car. Hate the drive to the nursing home.

I seem to be cursing, like a Tarratt Syndrome reaction to stress. F-this! F-that! F... F... F... Is there a medical condition of pronounced vulgarity related to unexpected situations of increased pressure to sustain a positive direction? No curve, no twist, no back peddling. Straight ahead. Damn!

Our visit was short. She said my touch helped her to sleep.

Hate the drive back to the house.

November 15th – Night.

I watch the night sky. A half-moon. Venus! A meteor shower scheduled. Power and consistent motion. No stars tonight. Light fog.

Her space in the nursing home is near the hallway door. The window is above the third bed. Out back a double row of motel rooms, bars on the windows. A patch of blue is visible.

Pills to soothe the pain and reduce the stress. Stress, needing a pill to ease pain. Pain, pill, pain, pill, pain.

Grow older, gracefully.

I remember poor Dotty. A friend.

The women exited Leisure World, the d.d. ran the light, killed the women – Dotty. I remember the funeral. I pray for her soul each night. Twelve years have passed.

Everyone knows someone harmed or killed in a highway tragedy – avoidable tragedy.

November 16th – Sunday Morning.

Visited for two hours. I took my wife a new picture of Madalyn Rose, our great-granddaughter, age five months. The baby is dressed in black and white harlequin tights and surrounded by pumpkins. Taped to the wall, she smiles at my wife.

We talked about my sister, she called from Oregon. Her son plans to join the Navy. Her oldest daughter has two and four year old children, boy and girl. Francis, the youngest daughter, is expecting. We had planned a trip to visit my sister in the spring. Perhaps next summer. Depending on recovery.

I read sea poems; she fell asleep. I remember reading my western novel to my friend, Lee, in a Hollywood nursing home; he fell asleep. Perhaps my writing needs more violence, more madness, more terror – more realism. More sex!

November 16th – Night.

Recovery slow; fatigue fast. Bellyache from fractured ribs, bruising. The battle injury, cracked rib from a fist or bat, fall off a cliff. In the soap opera the girlfriend touches the tender flesh, the winch. The kiss to soothe the pain.

Back to the nursing home where ordinary people stretch and groan, fighting to be well. Where sons and daughters visit and encourage and pray. The husband, the wife, forever in love. You will be home soon. Never doubt.

The worst is over. The surgery complete. No more I.V. No constant blip-blip recording vital functions. You can lift from bed. Slow and easy. Steady. No wobble or fall. Give yourself time. Slow and easy. Remember, drugs impair your physical control.

November 16th – Night Time Call.
"Scratcher won three dollars. Birthday ticket."
"You still got the luck."
"You picked the winner. Visited dinner room. Tailbone pain.

Eye doctor appointment tomorrow. E-I-B-O
My eye chart reads OW-E-UE."
"Honey, I love you."
"Drug hangover. Heparin shot to belly. Blood thinner."
"Honey, be brave."
"Weight. Gained two pounds."
"Sounds good, love."
"Night love."
Exchange kissing.

November 17th – Police Report.
I received the d.d. collision police report. Valeria provided the copy. My numbers are correct. Eight possible deaths. Three additional passengers in the d.d. car. Three passengers asleep during the smoke and double crash. Perhaps it was ectoplasm instead of smoke. A ghost in the car would be a more plausible explanation for the black-out of three healthy young male specimens. College identity speculation and rumor. Gang members? Rock stars?

Speculation on conversation after collision. "Listen, only a minute before cops come. You guys were asleep. Jolted awake after the second crash. Missed the collision.

Agreed. I do all the talking. Say nothing." Silent agreement. Speculation.

Group Dynamics postulates an absolute truth. The individual abandons their identity to conform to a collective demand. A bond is unconditional.

Sunday morning, the quiet traffic, her warmth. Bonding! Coffee alone. One more week. Back on track.

The Bridge of San Luis Ray. Who are the witnesses? Are they college students? Gang members! Lives with a future. Innocent! The neighbor's sons. Illegals?

My brother's keeper. Sue the blip-blip-blip-blip. Failure to stop a criminal act, compliance with a crime. F... F... F... F... the blip-blip-blip-blip. Witness?

"The bang, crash. I was squashed between you guys. He's spinning the wheel, roller-coaster-ride. Slam, bang. Spinning cars like tops. Wow. Great! Man. Crunch. A couple old ladies fucked up. This was a blast."

Shut-up, silencio!

Shaking a fist, despair. Forgive! Temporary inconvenience. Pain for the rest of her life.

Conviction! Ankle bracelet? Time in the slammer? Is the judge of the criminal court a compassionate man? Consider? A young man, a new chance, mercy. Old lady, drive defensively. The jails are crowded, unsafe. The young man made a mistake.

A joke over beers. The stitches like a snake. A tattoo for the circus lady. Photos on the internet.

November 18th – Phone, Lunch.

"Shots in belly, for blood thinning. Weighed – one pound gained.

Tired out, new pain pills.

Lunch cake, spice cake, butterscotch topping – tasted good.

Met Max, blind man. Seven year resident."

Voice ended.

"Sleep dearest, deep, deep, peaceful sleep."

Get busy. Copy papers, send ambulance papers, pictures, papers, papers. Pills, pain, progress slow. Shots in the belly. Ouch! No swearing. I felt weary, deeply tired, down to my bones.

Once we accept our physical limits, we go beyond them. New energy drink, new pill. New exercise technique. New food. Nano robots with battery packs in the bloodstream. Yoga!

Clean the Venetian blinds. Vacuum. Dinner sandwich – cheese. Coat hanger – 2. Drugs helped. I slept, o.k. Breakfast dry. Card for JoJo – 5. Bedroom drawers, left side, check book.

Max, the man in the wheelchair is blind. A resident of the nursing home for seven years. A nice man.

A state prisoner cost is $50,000 a year. Old Max depends on social security, substantially less than prisoner compensation.

Caring for my wife is costly. We have paid into the insurance system for over fifty years. Pity the money is spent on a fool's crime.

Mark Twain said, "When angry, count to four, when very angry, swear."

%%$##&()))*&&@@)((****&^%#$#@@!++(*&%

My wife's mother, Andra, was artistic – painted impressionistic landscapes. My wife refuses to acknowledge she inherited her mother's artistic talent. "Can't paint like mom or my sister." Her display for every holiday is a masterpiece. Dress style, jewelry – immaculate design. Marilyn Monroe grooming. Imaginative home decoration. My wife is an artist!

Buy the cane that won't fall down. Amazing the medical innovations to facilitate physical need.

Positive images. The smile of the baby, a picture of health. Reinforcing image of health. Birthday cards and get well cards. Ribbons and bows. Flowers. A champagne bottle shaped card.

My friend, Lee, died in a nursing home. He listened to books on tape – westerns. **Hondo**!

I gave a tape player to my wife with a Lilian Jackson Braun novel, **The Cat Who Said Cheese**. My mother's favorite author. Mystery, solved by Siamese cats and a billionaire bachelor in Moose County.

Note: send medical information to lawyer.

November 19th – Phone, Night.
"Remember, Avon Lady, call her. She sends well wishes.

Find Ruth's birthday present in shed – follow my directions, tomorrow morning."

I write a note.

"Ate dinner, even a quarter of the bread. Grapes.

Korean desert.

Purple grapes. Feel well, got my medicine.

Rick in John's house, birthday is the 16th. He left a card. Look in yesterday's mail or the box. No mail Veteran's Day. Get caught up with the mail. No Halloween decorations to take down. Pull chain on porch light to make light work.

Fast day. Got blankets clean.

Getting well, first priority. Channel surfing.

Won thirty cents at Bingo. Second prize. An hour. Then visited with Judy.

New roommate has t.v. on.

Call about dinner. Went to potty. Shower in morning. Exercise arm. Keeping the braces. Ribs are hurting. Messed up on medicine at noon. Now the schedule is mixed wrong again. Sleeping pills on time make me sleep. Screw up the medicine. Terrible. Since day one!

Getting up to go to bathroom. Uncomfortable in robe – everyone is dressed. Uncomfortable – one more week."

"One week, love."

November 20th – Sunday

Pad that emits electric charge to location of pain, rapid relief. Does the device work? Ask a football player? Pain relief. Smiles from the women in the t.v. ad.

My friend was in the nursing home ten years ago. Move someone in – move someone out. Lead by kind workers. Hard workers. Restricted to bed, he died of blood poisoning – sore infection.

My wife is using a cream to restrict the risk of bed sores. Scary. Weight loss. Scary. Belly pain. Scary. Damn! Damn! Damn!

November 21st – Nightmare.

She describes the crash vividly. She sees the crash in her mind, over and over.

The spinning, the wall crushing the car. Valeria, blood dropping from her mouth.

First impact the d.d. driver. Spin into the wall – crash, bounce. Spin two into the wall, smash – slide, grind, stop. Alive. Pain!

November 21ˢᵗ – Morning Phone Call.

"Find Ruth's gift.

Belt???

So tired. Noisy in hall. Drugs will make you tired. Plopped myself down. Ice pack on my belly. Can't keep my eyes open. Full day. Awaken in night. Felt so good. Now feel apart. Love you!"

Last night I spent two and a half hours coping paper, preparing required mail to send to medical insurance and ambulance. Copies for lawyer.

She will be home soon. Her arm is out of the sling. Limp, weak, no lifting, no force. Slow, slow gentle movements guided by therapist.

We are a wild race.

Our self-importance boldly portrayed on the W.W.W.

When we think, we think of our self first.

I don't ever want to live in a nursing home.

I don't ever want to live in a jail.

Do we have the free will to decide our destiny? Forced to drink, forced to party, forced to gamble, forced to take a part in the play? Perception management? Subliminal impressions? Brainwashing? Drink and drive a casual mistake, harmless.

My wife said she did not hate the drunk driver. She did not want the anger and hate in her heart. Negative thought does not help the healing process. She is a wise woman.

I want justice. When beauty is trampled, the beast pays. A recent report observed college party drinking increasing. One student responds, "Try to stop us, we'll drink more." One million students drink daily.

Rambling. Wheelchairs rolling. Bright sunny day. Crash on the 91. No t.v. crews. Too early. No pictures in the dark. Three car collision in a Construction Zone.

Trip to the nursing home, second and fifth signal, three men texting. Three men in a row. What's wrong with the women today? Three to one, first two miles. Girls you score.

Rambling memories.

November 21st – 2nd Phone Call Noon.
"Wayne said a prayer. Ruth just left. I have a csesar salad.
Didn't bring medicine at six o'clock. In coming call.
Don't hang up.
Ruth's birthday gift. Rain deer ornament. I can hear Mildred's voice.
I'll call a nurse for her. I'll call back later.
Love you sweetie."

If I say it won't be long, it will seem longer. You'll be home in no time. A few more days. Hours… We are lucky we have each other.

Watch the arm exercise, the movement gently and slowly, guided by her therapist – Mario. A young man with wife and six year old girl. My wife told him about her favorite coloring book for children and she gave him a copy of **Penny the Pink Cloud.**

November 22nd – Therapy Room
Two women rotate the pedals on the bike machine, moving the handlebars in a cycle.

A therapist guides a man up the stairs, learning to move up and down a stairway.

The walls show a blue sea, sky and clouds, seagulls. A work bench for exam papers and computer terminals. A collection of walkers. A woman learning the correct use of a walker.

A busy therapy room, the gymnasium.

I remember buying pillars and wire for my friend, Lee. A nursing home project. Wire sculpting. The rare time I witnessed excitement in his eyes. The look of adventure. He was planning to fashion a wire motorcycle. Memory and purpose, powerful motivation.

I recall the news print epitaph of a prominent philosopher that committed suicide. He said, at the age of 60 he had experienced everything life offered.

I know my wife would like to see Madalyn Rose graduate high school. I know I would.

November 23rd
"Morning sweetheart."

"Eating breakfast. I love to hear your voice. Valeria texted. Marilyn called and has to care for Little Ryner. She'll visit tomorrow. Wish Ruth a happy birthday. I was up at five, went to bathroom. My robe dipped in toilet and I put on a dirty one.

Anyway, I was awake on and off all night. Now, I'm tired.

Brace off arm, but I can't raise my arm. Love you, love you lots. My eyes hurt. Get Visine and lip gloss.

Tom called. Tom and Nick went deer hunting. Tom shot a deer. Hunting again next weekend. Snow. Easy to track. Sixteen degrees. Toes freezing. Minnesota chill.

Came and took blood-pressure – Victoria, my nurse. Two belly shots a day. Got meds after six. Next at nine o'clock. Sleep pill and morphine. Got my bed comfortable. Watch a show. Cable channel. Distraction. Little headache.

Maintenance came in and asked about air vents. Turned fan on, too cold.

Wait... A call
Call you back."

"Call at noon. Trip to Lawyer."
"Bye babe."
"Bye Love."
Kiss! Kiss!

My hand shakes when I return the phone to rest.

My busy, busy darling. Center stage, ready to stand alone.

Measure bathtub to see about the shower stool. Size to fit bathtub. Need stool to sit inside tub.

Seat cushion, check out chair.

The involvement to rehabilitate an injury is like a domino effect. Learn to exercise the arm, operate the bed, adjust the brace, shower stool…

Check pillow cost for Judy.

Hair shampoo

Notes…

November 24th – Phone Call Noon.

"Valeria has a new car – Camaro – white. Rusty, her mechanic, set-up a deal with a car dealership. Delivered from Temecula. She received insurance pay-off for the new vehicle. Right away. Calling the car Caucasian. White Lightning, rejected. No reference to booze.

Now, tests for additional injury.

Short pants, medium blouse, I need in the morning.

Love you, just plop down. Wolfed down lunch.

The medicine to increase appetite works. Pickled cucumber. I love. Beef stroganoff.

Energy food. Gaining weight.

Love you, talk in an hour. Careful driving.

Kiss, love, kiss."

No change to her rough, gravelly voice. What happened to the sound I remember? A clear, lithe with the spark of laughter. Ask doctor?

Today, my wife and her gambling partner, Valeria, were scheduled for a free trip to Laughlin, Nevada. They have Diamond Status at the casinos, lucky players. I planned walking on the beach working on my sea poems. Canceled. I'm buying a seat for the shower. My bride trying to move her arm. I'll see her soon.

We enjoy life. Retirement is rare in our families. Death precedes retirement, usually.

We kiss all day. And, have whoopee anytime we desire. I miss the kisses. The touch of flesh. We kiss at the nursing home – hospital taste. At home, her lips are sweet. No sex for the immediate future – too much pain and possible irritation to the injuries.

Silly morning arguing about where the check-book is hidden. In the jewelry drawer. Check in the back. Look! Bills do not stop when misfortune strikes. They increase!

Ambulance payments. Please verify approval. Original approval letter lost.

The writing must wait. Tough to balance work and helping my wife. Retired, sharing work, life becomes easier. Now, the simple tasks we shared, laundry, vacuum, cooking, watering the flowers – solo chores. My wife is a hard worker. Retirement depends on financial circumstance. Excessive medical expense was not a part of our retirement plans.

November 26th – Night Phone.
"Hi Honey,"
"Valeria on the phone. Call you back."
"Ok. Bye."

Her voice guarded, why?

My wife said, someday, she and Valeria will blubber together. Not now. My tears are frequent.

I received her clothes from the collision. The jeans and blue sweatshirt cut to pieces. No more sleeves. No more pant legs. Cut away. Capable hands, trained operation, human magnificence, saving a life. God Bless every soul that touched my darling. God Bless their loved ones now and forever.

The moon will be full before she comes home. Time is moving fast. Ten days on a catheter, twenty days in diapers, and now the toilet with an ingenious lift seat for unbendable limbs. Medical marvels.

The blind man and the wandering mystic passed room 14A and greeted my wife. "Calamity survivors touch heaven, have long life lines," the psychic lady told my wife. A happy thought. Life expectancy 107.

Skeletal support pants with computer control was demonstrated on television. Perfect for Judy, her knees are bad. The timetable of events, the last generation to die. The future plan, download Mr. Potter's brain into the quantum computer and download the electronic duplication into a fresh clone. Age twenty-seven was the desired model. Da, Da – Dm, Dm. Twilight Zone.

November 26th – Phone Call Back.

"Hi Honey,"

"When Marilyn came, we were out on the patio. Really beautiful out there."

"We need to fix the washing machine."

"More arm therapy, afternoon, walking exercise."

"Under a week."

"The dementia patient is talking. She has a loud, projecting voice.

Sister was here a couple hours.
Still two shots for blood thinning.
I love you.".
"I'm reading a James Bond novel; he has to stop a war."
"Anyway, I'm going to get comfortable."
"Bye, love you, bye love."

In chapter one Bond meets a woman surprisingly similar to my wife. Nordic, blue eyes, blond, curvaceous figure, beautiful smile. Vital!

Slip back to yesterday. Before the scar, her smile, laugh, energy. Now, a new face, skeletal, the eyes glitter green, burning. Pictures from yesterday, rosy cheeks, sparkly hair, her new style (her sister is a master beautician) now strains of straw, sweat bonding a gray streak to her brow.

Grow older gracefully. Ten years older in a heartbeat. God Bless you baby.

Escape destruction. There is a story I was told by a survivor. The Candy Broker. Plane crash lands on Salt Lake City airport runway. The plane an inferno. He escaped. The man beside him was a professional wrestler. The wrestler could not move his body. Frozen panic. The stewardess helped an older lady escape, and went back in the plane to help. The Candy Broker escaped with a broken back. Survival. One freeze. One hero. One with miraculous power.

I freeze in emergency. During the Big Bear Quake in 1992 (7.6) I turned white, was unable to move. Stuck on the stairway swaying like on a stormy sea. Frozen panic.

Of course, there is the coward or cowards.

I cannot damn the cowards for a lie. I cannot forgive. Impossible to forget. I comprehend the concept of justice. Is there any legal penalty for participating with the d.d. Knowingly going along with criminal action. The witnesses saw the d.d. drinking at the party. The witnesses accompanied the d.d. in the car, knowing a crime is in progress. The witnesses handed the d.d. the key. The witnesses are accomplices in the crime. Willing participants, allowing the d.d. to fire the gun. Compliance to a crime, a warning to every passenger, anyone willing to ride with a d.d.

November 27th – Night Phone.

"Hi handsome,"

"Hi darling."

"Call you right back. There's a baggy on the floor. I don't want anyone to slip on it.

I need to call someone. Call you right back."

Pause. Ring-ring.

"Hi baby."

"Peanut butter cookie in a bag. The bag fell. Called out a nurse. Didn't want any slip.

Marilyn left and Elaine came.

On one birthday card – one word comes to mine – Charming! Neat card.

One card is a character from a show and a bracelet cutout.

Nice visit for a long afternoon.

Dinner was good. Leafy salad. Italian dressing. Tasty.

Wayne and Gail stopped by. Always appreciate the prayer and they make a nice couple.

My nose keeps itching.

Love you, good night."

"Love you, sweet dreams."

Short ride in a fast lane. Back again tomorrow.

Three quarter moon. The rabbit running up the hill.

Starlight, star bright, please grant a wish tonight. Healing power and strength for my wife.

She will be home on Tuesday. Slow and gentle. Every step, new.

I moved the glass cabinet out of the bedroom. The bedroom is the #1 location for falls. No glass. Cushions along the wall.

Clear hallway, clear bathroom. No rugs. Buy rubber pad slipper socks. Bubble wrap hip belt?

It isn't seeing something new. It's seeing something there you missed before. You always loved her. On sight, the New Year Eve at the party on the Queen Mary. We shared a glass of champagne. Danced. A kiss at midnight. Next day I phoned. I love her voice.

The harm we inflict by misjudged behavior. Pain.

The prisoners await execution. $100,000 a year jail cells. Too dangerous to co-exist with prisoners outside death-row. Brother, sister, father, mother, uncle, son, aunt – hear the collective moan. Ghosts in shadows, criminally insane. A lifetime commitment to provide a home. No choice. The State cannot execute.

Fixated on the backyard fence. Street gang drunks easy excess, easy escape. Property defense limited. State laws. Pepper spray for the retired, aged.

November 28th – Morning Phone Call.
"Woke up at four. Can't sleep. Exhausted. Noise.

Different environment. I can't sleep.

I want to bend my knee and can't. Just feeling uncomfortable.

I'm eating my breakfast.

Just feeling over tired.

I'll feel better after a shower."

The hoarse voice keeps bothering me.

"Check suitcase. Check pants and blouse. Make-up lotion. Little white flat bottle. I need the lotion.

Check back before you come visit."

"Just called to cheer you up, honey. I love you."

"Waiting for rehab session.

A weirdo day. Tired! Different state of mind, slow motion. A morphine high. Time released. Zapped in E.R.

Think, knowing I'm going home. I'm getting anxious. A long, high hill to climb.

Hot day. Wash floor.

Just keep working. Squeeze the penguin.

Ok. Love you. Bye. Call back soon.

Love you."

Her voice, pain!

Morning news, plane crash. Survivors interviewed. Immediate attention. Front page news. Witness the result. Take a long look. Remember. Pain.

Drunk driving crash. A day on the freeway in Southern California. Common! No death. No news. A part of life. A drunk party, captain crashing the boat into the jetty – caption with picture – three dead. Young baseball star killed.

Who cares? Passengers and drivers killed every year. The families care. A loved one damaged beyond repair. The hard reality of disfigurement. A mind unbalanced. Nightmares. The scars. Pain…

Rehearsal for the final hour. Seven o'clock call. I should drive the night traffic, visit her bedside. Traffic is maddening. Street repair, digging a trench three miles along the route.

Silly explaining. My sweetheart is in a trance. Slave to pain. Now, chaotic calls from her delusional roommate.

People suffer. The death-pill, right-to-choose, a practical approach to the here-after.

Give the death-row prisoners a bottle of here-after pills. Free choice.

November 29th – Night Phone.

The moon is grown full faster than my wife's recovery. Smiles, discharge in three days, earlier than predicted.

Tomorrow, clothes selection. Grocery – rolls for more sandwiches – cheese and ham.

Ring-Ring-Ring

"Hello darling." I listened. I love her voice.

"Ruth visited. Late night therapy. A new girl worked my arm. Twenty minutes for good arm. Walk the stairs; walk around the building.

Tomorrow I'll need clothes.

Also, credit card for hospital bed. Tomorrow, Friday, I'll set-up the hospital bed delivery.

Hamburger, plain, a cup of dressing. Too dry.

Settle in – ready for bed. No use of arm. Careful. No movement. Really. Let them do the movement. Really, really watch myself.

JoJo called and thanked us for birthday card.

Talked to Daisy. Sisters are special.

Doctor approved new prescription when I leave.

I love you."

"Soon, baby, soon."

"At home, I have to do a lot of walking.

Anyway, I'll call you before bedtime.

Ok."

"Yes darling, I love you. Love, love, love you."

I'll never hear a sig-alert without hearing pain, a siren seared in my brain.

A time of joy, my wife walking, coming home in three days. Yet, I'm moaning and groaning about the financial situation. On a fixed income, giving more than receiving becomes costly. Our gift to the grand-children, a day at Disneyland, maximum interest on the credit card charge. Mr. Disney, what happened to fair play – 9.9% is Uncle Sam's rate, outrageous. Greed!

Immediate expense like the gas to the nursing home add-up fast. Where do all the tax dollars go, forty cents for every gallon worth of gas goes to the government. Wow! One week take, I could build a nursing home on the moon. Near weightless environment would help Judy recover her knee strength, possibly.

November 30th – Noon Phone.

Ring-Ring

"Hi Honey, Just a second. I'm having lunch. I'll call you back."

"Take your time, dear."

Ring-Ring

"Lunch… two chicken thighs, corn bread, zucchini and pears for desert. All kinds of good stuff. I've been eating well."

Exciting, good feeling. Stop to think where we were this month a year ago. Travel plans. Remember… This month was surreal. Only to become better.

"Carlos delivered medicine. Handsome young man, blue scrubs, smile. Checked blood sugar. Index most punctured. Use the middle finger. Heparin shots for blood thinning.

Percocet 10-3-2-5

10 is dosage – 3-2-5

9:00 a.m. – 9:00 p.m. Morphine

Walked outside.
Smell the roses."
"I love you very much."
"I love you. Step by step."

Idea for a Reality T.V. Show – Nursing Home Survival. Or, Reality Show – Prison Madness. No contest. Fist fights verses palates exercise. Tattoo verses scar. Young, tough verses older, feeble. Healthy verses injured. Dark verses light. The devil will always win top billing in Hollywood. **Highway to Heaven** represents the exception.

Alignment of date numbers like the years my wife explained about birthdates. One hundred years after Ruth's birthday, good date to reincarnate. Alaska! Curious, abstract alignment. Numerologists could explain the D.U.I. collision. 0-chaos, confusion. 1-creation, order, reason. 2-duality, conflict, division. 3-divinity, realization. 4-squarness, justice, mystery. 5-fullness of life, exuberance. 6-adjustment to material conditions. 7-peace, completeness, satisfaction. 8-friendship, material perfection. 9-intuition, inspiration, drama. Retirement = 777. D.U.I. = 000

Invalid, scary to think the word. A chronically sick or disabled person.

Our neighbor's dog barks every night for hours. Neighbors are tolerant.

My wife will welcome the noise. A familiar home serenade. And, she will never again complain about the scout ants in the bathtub. The squeaky door hinge – music.

December 1st – Night Phone.
Ring. Ring.
"Hi Honey."
"Just a second. I'm having my dinner. I'll call you back."

"Take your time, dear."

Tenseness in our afternoon visit. Missing paper, argument.

Pain... Diary of a Highway Victim – Drunk Driver Collision

Arguments and frustration. "Find the sweat-shirt with the Glacier logo in the bag by the shoes. No! Too the right of the shoes. Look, are you blind."

Feeling tired. Phone ringing a third time. Three tries – new rule, call back time – ten minute max. Ring-ring.

"Hello dear, talking to Valeria."

"Ok. I've been calling. I'm going to bed. Tired. Say hello to Valeria. I love you. You sound good."

"I love you. Sleep well, dear."

"Tomorrow, love."

Read, distraction, sleep. Headache. Bond, James Bond visiting the nursing home on the big screen in the dinning room. Coincidental. **Goldfinger**. My book is by a new author, British. Bond is 45, the year 1969, African civil war. Sound familiar. We all know Bond has suffered pain. Lucky in love. A drinking man. 007 forever!

A powerful distraction. Double damn! Frustration and fatigue. A curious blend to elicit depression. Write another page. For my darling suffering a million times my weakly, wimpy headache.

December 2nd – Morning Phone.

"Hello sweetheart."

"Sweetheart. Feeling tired.

Phone ringing at three.

Talking all night.

Need a wake-up pill.

Eating breakfast – Belgium waffle with sugar free cereal. With cranberry juice. Mocha mix, don't like, tastes like coffee. Out of water.

Find clothes.

Constipation problem.

Wish I had another pair of sweatpants. Color gray. The sweats go over the brace. And, another blouse. Tomorrow, we have to call for the hospital bed. We need bars for the tub with suction. Something to consider. The therapist said the suction bars work well. Things we need to get.

Hour, get back to me. I love you. Ok."

Radio noise deadens loneliness.
Crash!
Lanes backed-up
Pain!
A mess on the 60
Crash on the 55
Sig-alert
Motorcycle down.
Injury! Injury! Injury!
Pain! Pain! Pain!
D.U.I. or Texting
Damn! Damn! Damn!

Imagery, a word picture, defines poetry – Ezra Pound. The mind flashes on multiple images in a moment. The bookcase, window pane, hummingbird, desk lamp, black and blue torso… Anterior cingulate cortex – emotions triggered by pain.

Positive images are posted on the walls above the beds in the nursing home. People pictures, memories, bows, hearts, cards… The reminders of love. A distraction from pain. Balloons! The mind never forgets the images.

December 3rd – Visit to Bedside

"Nurse, I like, gave me a good dinner. Apple juice, cheese ravioli, big round noodles, cheesy, delicious, tasty. And, garlic on bread toast.

I have a list of groceries for when I get home. Ruth, cooking up a turkey for us. She's visiting her friend in Las Vegas.

Anxious. Six o'clock meds. Top – short sleeve shirt purple and gray. Don't forget.

Tailbone pain is misery. Rib pain is misery. Dry mouth. Tired.

Undress, I'll be careful."

I fluff her pillows. Kiss her lips.

"One girl knows how to fluff pillows. I'll take her home with me. We have pillows packed away. Allergy free. Hospital bedding, Misty finding bedding. She bought and washed bedding.

Leather chair, put chair outside. Cover up. Good idea. Room for hospital bed. Sorry, I'm not tucking you in bed. I love you. Sweet dreams.

We'll clear out stuff tomorrow.

Love you."

I leave her softly dreaming. Wrinkles of pain on her face.

Note: Names…

Courtney and sister Gabby, nurses dispense medicine.

J.R. dispenses medicine.

Mildred – makes bed.

Dennis – helps serve.

Ernesto – therapist

April – the social worker.

Caynelle and Crisiant – therapists.

Aeesha – nurse aid and past student.

Brought ice pack on visit. "This stinks," my wife complained. Wrong ice pack. I brought a package of salmon.

Greatest triumph; greatest sorrow. Love! Evasive. Smoldering. Magical. Love. A tender flower, raging river – love. A gift to ease the pain – love.

Where is the villain, now? His friends, watching football, gulping beer, chomping popcorn. Too young for bars. Borders closed. New party house, not far from home.

"He was a fool."

"He should have known better."

"Idiot."

"First offense!"

"College student?"

"Crowded jails."

"Bracelet, my bet."

"Bet five on the blue team."

"You're on."

December 3rd – Night

Calling for our good-night kiss. Another night alone.

A bright night. A full moon. Clouds flowing over the moon, wisps of white. My darling covered with soft sheets tonight. With puffy pillows.

Pixie balloons to lift her arm and rest her weary back. Quiet, peace. Sweet dreams dearest.

I remember reading **The Bridges of Madison County** and crying. Love is a force, powerful like the moon gravity rolling the ocean tides.

A war photographer. The country wife. Simple people. Peaceful, simple people, untouched by the world racing around. I wish the nursing home patients peaceful dreams. Peaceful life. Peaceful death.

My sister said she saw the light and more. She was hit in the head in a rock fight in the riverbed. She was a tom-girl, older sister. She saw the tunnel of light and at the end of the light a Woman, long white hair, a tiny lady. "You don't belong here." A mental message. Presto, my sister was back in the sand pile, bleeding, aware of a timelessness and the impeccable knowledge of heaven. She told me.

What was the song name – **Heaven Is In Your Mind.** Sis said she had never seen the lady, all dressed in white, anytime before in her life. Who can tell? Life and death – mysteries. Sad to die because of stupidity. Especially the stupidity of a complete stranger. A gun accident hunting – acceptable. Blind sided by a drunk – stupid death.

December 4th – Morning Phone

"Gail and Wayne visited last night. Wayne prayed for me.

Didn't go anywhere. Lying in bed. The noise is amazing. Patients screaming. Doing construction. Refurbishing a room down the hall. They start work at sun-up. Carpenter cowboys.

Oh look.

Judy and Shirley are here. I'll let you go. I love you."

Can you picture the stage play? The dignity of age, stripped to diapers and socks. Plastic knifes and spoons. The donut toss, instead of pillows. Wheel chair whirling, crutches ka-wack, the drumbeat of feeble hearts.

The D.U.I. collision survivor leaves tomorrow.

Which one?

The psychic lady spoke to my wife last night. She was excited about the little baby born with the gastroschisis condition. "Survivors off rare complications are rewarded with rare gifts. The child is blessed. I will visit her and give her a special power. Tonight, I will leave my body and travel to her bedside. She is special."

My wife was pleased by the words, however the visit mention was perplexing. Astro-projection, the psychic lady explained. Soul travel!

December 5th – Night Phone
"Hi Honey."
"Hi Babe.

Waiting for dinner. Fish again with white rice, zucchini, cranberry juice. Not suppose to eat white rice. Watching **Adam-12**. Cable hook-up. Adventure channel. 300 selling channels.

Old time set, twenty-two inch screen. We need to measure. Old t.v. with thick back.

Few more days. Doing the whoopy. Tonight, next pills 9:00 o'clock, off to dreamland.

Saturday night.

Now a baking show, about cup cakes.

Visited on the patio during exercise. Getting cool. My room is warm. Quieted down, still noisy. Activities started at 2:30. Judy won two bingo games – she won 30 cents.

I'm going to go to the bathroom.

Call, I love you.

Kiss... Bye!"

Drive home, radio...
Traffic Alert
7 car collision

3 critical injuries
D.U.I. arrest…

December 6th – Phone Dinner.
"How you doing?"
"Just got tired. Kinda bored. Just finished dinner. More fish for dinner and macaroni. Tilapia fish. You know the kind we like.

Soup for lunch, peas, very good.

Maintenance crew working on the leak. Drip! Drip! Drip! Drip! All last night. Drip in the middle of the room. Soaking the middle bed. I have to get out of here.

Now, I'm comfortable.

Asked for blanket and sheet. For tonight. Good to look ahead. Takes a while to receive things.

I need to know about the back pain from walking. And, make sure about the blood thinner. I have notes on the telephone.

Weighed me on gurney.

Talked to Marilyn.

Didn't lose anymore weight. The brace gives wrong numbers. Can't tell real weight.

My back hurts after a walk. More pain, sweetheart. Complaining. Love you so much.

Get back to you in the morning.

Too-da-loo-da. Love you, bye."

Sunday. Rain possible. Our California weather reporters sometimes exaggerate rainy conditions.

A drop of rain hit my head. One drop. In California, six raindrops colliding make a storm.

The moon is full. Shock, a mild tremor. Turmoil. Depressed. Call. List for tomorrow. Night. Fatigue. Write.

No novel, or play. I always wanted to write – non-stop, the words tumbling out, like Jean Paul Sartre locked in a room – **Being and Nothingness**.

No masterpiece, the **Quran**.

No plot, a collection of characters without significant quality, no bigger than life image – normal people. The refugees of age and desire. A diary. Teenage girl obsession replaced by face book.

The rambling of an old man. The thread weaved through the pages – misery. Hope!

December 7th – Morning Phone.

"Morning, darling."

"Love you."

"Bad night. Sleeping pill, no help. **Revenge** was on at 9:00. Thirty six hour count down.

Tom – no luck hunting.

Ruth's birthday just passed. Want a laugh. Next year, month, day, Tom's birthday is dated in number sequence with Ruth's date. Won't happen again for a century."

Third repeat of same message. Drugs… Pain… A mantra for positive energy?

"I'm back. Love you. Love you.

Didn't do anything about the drip.

Carlene, the nurse, is really named Mildred. Nice young woman. She has two small children – boy and girl.

The new woman sharing the room talks and talks. *Santa Anita noon sweepstakes. Filly, old nag, Grasshopper, blue flag, blue fag. A million to one, old roster crow, ding-dong. Winner.* She must be visiting the racetrack in her mind. Reliving a horse race.

Lord Jesus, bless and ease her troubled mind.
Breakfast is here. Call back.
Love you. Bye."

The Countdown: 36 hours.

Consolidated alignment – Venus meets the moon. You spent all night racing past. A special night. Star cluster beyond Sirius, seven earth planets discovered. Sweet surrender. The soul leaving the old home.

Pearl Harbor Remembrance Day. War veterans remembered. Madness and pain. Premeditated pain and blind direction. Painful memories of needless destruction. The year 2000 – enlightenment. Silly idea. We're only human. The march for peace is slow and long, abused by false circumstance. Pray for peace.

December 8th – Full Moon.

The d.d. must be thankful he didn't kill someone that morning. He must be smart to concoct a smoke story minutes after the collision. Many intelligent people – neighbors and friends – thrive in America. Intelligence does not beget common sense and common sense begets wisdom. Time and reflection, a straight path. "Youth is wasted on youth." Who said that? "Common sense is as rare as genius." Who said that?

My wife will walk with pain. Live with pain. Die in pain.
He will live behind bars?
Guilty and Innocent.
The punishment.
Criminal Trial – 63 days.

********* ********** ********* ********

IX

Third Letter to Our Lawyer

Dear Lawyer:

Sincere apology for my stubborn attitude and lack of legal comprehension. After review of the clear and objective advice on recent phone counsel, we will continue to prepare for a Civil Trial. Enclosed is a check for five thousand dollars. Our commitment to "fairness and respect" for the victim and the most severe judgment for the criminal D.U.I. is the same for the Civil Trial as it is for the Criminal Trial. Hopefully, the Civil Trial will favor the "seriously injured" passenger.

The older body is slower to repair with more painful complications. Currently and for the foreseeable future my wife experiences knee pain walking. Chest pain – eating. Arm pain – persistent. Back pain! Fatigue from medication and pain. Once she was a busy women into midnight. Now she is asleep by nine. Estimated four hours of her normal day gone. Considering severity of injury and age of victim, struggle to heal is testament to women's courage.

My wife continues medical treatment for injuries from the D.U.I. collision on October 20th. Test for chest pain scheduled. Scheduled knee surgery will hopefully eliminate pain. Serious back pain. Back surgery scheduled. Doctors cannot find reason for sweats and chills. Before the collision her weight was over 140 pounds, now under 110 pounds. 120 pounds is medically acceptable. Pain management therapy – next step. A struggle to maintain the delicate balance to avoid increased pain. "I need to lie down. Dizzy!" Repeated daily. How fragile she has become in such a short time.

Victims requested maximum penalty for D.U.I. collision on October 20th in a Construction Zone. Eight people in a deadly collision. To deter future D.U.I. crime the severest penalty is justified. The Criminal Court is lenient. A recent Olympic Champion received a 2nd D.U.I. speeding 40 miles over the posted limit, weaving over the yellow line, twice the legal alcohol level in his blood. Judgment broadcast to every sports fan in every bar in the U.S.A. One and a half years of probation. The poster-boy for D.U.I. No harm, no crime.

Minimum coverage from Progress D.U.I. insurance and zero coverage from Multi-State insurance for passenger in vehicle totaled. Infinite, zero response. No reference to D.U.I. criminality in the policies. A series of letters to insurance and probation department shows a lack of concern for D.U.I. passenger victim.

Request for D.U.I. policy #0000000-0; zero acknowledgement from Progress.

Request for D.U.I. driving history to confirm "reckless" driving charge. No response. D.U.I. insurance repair of collision vehicle and current driving status of D.U.I. teen.

Information withheld. Request to court for criminal history of D.U.I. No response. Request for D.U.I. policy or "mission statement" from insurance agencies. Nothing! Request for example of "high risk" insurance policy. Nothing!

Requests for information with SASE addressed to victim returned with no response. Restriction of information to the victim on the basis of legal representation is a legal principle we are ignorant of violating. We are simply interested in information to decide to proceed to a Civil Trial. Also, the question of responsible insurance for teen drivers with "reckless" record. Insurance Commissioner letter response enclosed. Your name was not included in the correspondence.

We hope we haven't caused any serious trouble by requesting D.U.I. information. The information was requested to determine a decision to proceed to Civil Trial. We informed the correspondent the information would be discussed with our lawyer. Possibly the information requests are in your files – drunk driver's insurance policy, driving record, and criminality status – please mail copies to our address.

Information leads to a clear and complete picture of a subject; a principle followed by high school educators. Obviously, personal information is confidential. However, the state requires motorist insurance and the insurance agency D.U.I. policy or Mission Statement should be public record. Three powerful insurance agencies – Multi-State and Progress and Infinite – unwilling to provide a statement to a concerned motorist about a very common highway tragedy – D.U.I. collision.

The complete lack of D.U.I. reference in insurance policies is disturbing. Policy of all insurance agencies guaranteeing insurance coverage to passengers willingly and knowingly driven by a drunk driver is very disturbing. And, the persistent protection of the D.U.I. criminal by multiple insurance agencies is very, very disturbing. Accountability by the d.d. criminal participants and insurance agency cannot be ignored by judge and jurors.

On the positive side, perhaps the letters to three insurance representatives influenced the resent news report that insurance agencies might increase insurance coverage for teen divers – report on radio. Progress and Multi-State insurance agencies are defending a teen limited policy acknowledged by the insurance industry as inadequate to reflect the serious lack of driving safety in teen drivers. Increased insurance coverage for "reckless" motorists and convicted "D.U.I." motorists is next step to protect honest motorist from dangerous drivers.

The insurance agency with statistical knowledge of the potentially dangerous drivers, should be held accountable for providing inadequate insurance coverage for teens, "reckless" drivers and "D.U.I." criminals. The teen was allowed to buy minimum insurance despite knowledge of negative teen driving statistics and common sense insurance proposals to require increased insurance policy coverage for teens. A teen with "reckless" driver charge allowed minimum insurance coverage is wrong. Substandard business practice by insurances providers is evident.

Defending the limited D.U.I. teen insurance policy while preparing to require increased teen coverage is hypocritical. Insisting "reckless" driving requires no additional insurance is wrong. The insurance agencies have had full knowledge of the statistical predicable consequence involving teen drivers for many years. In the near future all insurance agencies will support the higher insurance requirement for teen drivers. The insurance agencies knew of the teen lack of coverage on October 20th and kept the facts suspended like the auto company recently guilty of hiding the faulty part while drivers died. Lack of value for human life.

Our resolve to hold the D.U.I. and the D.U.I. representative responsible for a reasonable settlement for the "seriously bodily injury" of senior citizen passenger victim is firm. Maximum penalty possible in Civil Trial. Probably, a child's loss of arm function and pain involving a longer life results in a higher insurance settlement. The Criminal Trial judgment must be seriously committed to punish the drunk driver responsible for eight near deaths in an explosive collision in a Construction Zone.

Considering the current insurance settlement will not provide the cost to repair dental damage, the Civil Court is the only option for reasonable settlement and insurance guarantee for future medical expense resulting from the D.U.I. collision. At present we assume no insurance challenge is considered by the insurance agencies against injured victim's right to Handicap Space. Possibly in Civil Court with insurance doctors and insurance lawyers, the Handicap Sticker will be revoked. The policy of a fixed settlement for all injury is unfair, especially when the injury is criminally inflicted by an identified dangerous motorist.

The D.U.I. is free. An average American yearly income requires hard work and discipline. The d.d. teen has no car expense. Rental and food cost minimum. Unemployment is 5%. An honorable and hard worker – the financial possibilities in America are unlimited. "Fairness and respect" for the victim is the path to acquittal for the act of violence. Perhaps the Civil Court can offer Caltrans work and a long term lone to pay the victim's settlement. In the Criminal Trial Caltrans often provide the criminal D.U.I. an alternative from a possible lose of freedom.

Financial compensation for D.U.I. Civil Trial legal defense is guaranteed by D.U.I. insurance policy. However, using money collected from the convicted D.U.I. criminals to defend future D.U.I. criminals is a questionable practice. Financial compensation for victim's legal assistance is not guaranteed by the court or victim's insurance, unfortunately. Hopefully, the Civil Court will help the victim of the D.U.I. The passive approach to D.U.I. criminality is unacceptable.

Reduction of legal cost was considerate, especially appreciated by fixed income retirees. Monetary compensation for an ill deed is legal tradition. Legal counsel guarantee of 40% of the Civil Trial returns is secondary to establishing common sense law – "reckless" and "D.U.I." motorists require "high risk" insurance – and sending a clear message to four party drunks that demolition derby in a Construction Zone is a violent, premeditated atrocity. Every possible deterrent and protection against D.U.I. is the goal of every honest motorist. D.U.I. crime is 100% preventable.

God Bless the Highway Victims.
Respectfully,

The Highway Victim

********** ********** ********** **********

X

Victim's Impact Statement – Judge Letter

ORANGE COUNTY PROBATION DEPARTMENT
VICTIM IMPACT STATEMENT

****

Defendant's Name: Xxxx   ML# A000000

Case # 00NR00000   Court Date: XX/00/0000   Incident Date: 10/20/0000

***** ***** ***** *****

Name of Victim of the D.U.I. Collision: (Name)

Date of Birth: 00/00/0000 Features: blue-eyed, blond, beautiful Retired County Worker

Children: 2   Grandchildren: 6   Great-grandchildren: 1   Husband: (Name)

***** ***** ***** *****

LETTER FOR THE JUDGE:

Diary: December 8, 0000

Wake-up one morning with pain equivalent to severe bursitis – shoulder, neck, arm. Back ache/Knee pain/Belly ache. Weighed against an outcome of eight dead, the devil lost! The mark of the battle scars my wife, but Angels guard her sleep.

Scary to see weak health. Suffering. Walking a tightrope, fragile balance. Pain inescapable. She is brave, she strains to regain top health, endures the pain. We guard against additional harm. No lifting. Stay warm. Rest. Light exercise. Return to day-to-day activity with limitation – arm, leg, back, ribs.

Left arm, no power, no lifting, constant pain. Back ache and knee pain increase with movement. Ribs healing. Lethargic, sleep time excessive. Weight loss, muscle loss, skin wrinkle. Rosy vitality turned to weakness and pallor. No snuggling, no hugging, no spooning. Moans, groans, whimpers – new sounds in our home.

Gentle cuddle and kisses. She is always my beautiful bride. God bless her.

My lawyer instructed us to write a diary. 20,000 words since the D.U.I. collision, one message repeated over and over – the curse of unwanted pain!

Eight humans escaped death on October 20, 0000. The car my wife's friend was driving was totaled. The quick, correct actions of emergency personnel rescued my wife and her friend. My wife will live with unwanted pain, increasing in intensity with the aging process, for the rest of her life.

Three car insurance companies are involved in compensation for medical costs. Fortunately, my wife, a retired county worker, is medically insured. However, hospital reimbursement is being requested. And, orthopedic apparatus and additional therapy treatment is still questionable. Time expended on recovery – every hour, every day.

Future medical expense – ramps, rails, wheelchair – is unpredictable. I have an annuity saved from my teaching salary for emergency. We have fixed incomes. Our retirement business speculation – writing and selling a book for language improvement

English/Spanish Crossover Diccionario – has been suspended. A second book of poetry with illustrations by my mother-in-law, publication postponed. My wife is my proofreader and #1 fan. I am a lexicographer because of her support and help.

My darling wife endures constant pain. Sometimes she has a look in her eyes like a child after unexplained punishment, wondering what she did wrong. Health is the treasure of greatest value. My wife spent over a month in hospital and nursing home. A plate of metal is screwed into her shoulder, a scar slash with 42 staple points. Home recovery is slow, painful. Worry and fear a new headache.

The medical condition of my wife continues to be analyzed and treated. Her state of health, once life threatening, now stable. A fall could send her back to the nursing home. Drugs, weakness, pain. A radical change in our retirement dream.

Eight people in a D.U.I. collision. Death is final! What is the message to college students accused of increased drinking activities in recent years? Party until dawn! Friends drive drunk! I believe the d.d. is a coward. I believe he was running away when he hit the second car, slamming the car into a concrete wall – twice. His friends, remain silent – cowards. They pay no penalty for allowing a d.d. to drive – compliance to a crime. Three peaceful sleepers through two metal bashing impacts.

The collision report is a competent and complete record of the D.U.I. crime. We met Officer X.X. Xxxxxx (ID #00000) in the hospital, a conscientious and considerate California Highway Patrol Officer. The recommended punishment by M.A.D.D. for like D.U.I. collisions will be acceptable justice. M.A.D.D. common punishment consensus for similar crimes – driving twenty miles above the speed limit in a Construction Zone, intoxicated from an all night party, smashing two cars, totaling one, emergency room injuries, permanent physical damage.

Restitution? Recently a basketball star was sentenced to three years probation for D.U.I. If he were hit by a drunk driver like my wife, he would have a career ending injury. My wife shoots hoops and bounces the basketball with the grandchildren on special occasions. Rayette, granddaughter, is a star basketball player in high school. We attend her graduation in June; she enters a Christian college in the fall. Ask the three passengers in the car with the d.d. the value of their arms? Priceless!

We recently received the title of great-grandparents. Madalyn Rose born last year, June 1st, a gastroschisis baby. We are grateful for the miracle of life.

God bless the people that helped my wife survive the D.U.I. collision. God bless the eight survivors. Good Health and Long Life.

Respectfully,

Name of Victim

Orange County Court
State of California
XX/00/0000

********** ********** ********** **********

XI

Diary – Home Rehab

December 9th – Phone Night.

"Called to say good-night. I love you. Call in the morning. Sweet dreams. Tired…"

Whispered words. No hospital bed delivery until after 8:00 at night. Can't wait till morning. Original time was 2:00 to 6:00. The irritations multiply with pain. Morose emotional status. The high and low, elated and tired shift in mood is not normal for my wife. Anger leads to harm. Damn!

A voice screaming in this wilderness. A meaning to life. Her face in the mirror. A teardrop. Yesterday's blemish. Go forward bravely.

Last ten days, $150 million for a movie previews. The drip-drip of a leak, the last straw, a Chinese torture technique. No, the frustration of too little for too many. The profit motive, compassion and diligence secondary. Pay less, get more. Rolling in the weak, out go the well. Business is booming. Low overhead.

Picked up a present. Gave my wife a whistle. When she needs assistance, she blows the whistle and I jump to her call.

What's wrong with taking life for granted. Home sweet home. Trivial pursuit. Paint the garage trim. Watch the tit-bird dive for supper. Her soap opera. My poetry. First step for Madalyn Rose.

Now what do we do? Sex with pain. Whips and chains. God forbid! Easy does it every time. Gentle touch, the wounded bride.

When a sparrow flies into a window, snaps the wingtip. The cat cares. Sparrows are common. The brains tasty. Thank God her brains were spared.

Nursing home residents. The sense of acceptance. Man with broken leg. Lady on crutches. The mother of two daughters, living for the next visit, white hair, white skin, delicate. Arms in slings, necks in braces, knee splints, swaths of bandage. A weary pace. Age the greatest burden. The failure of a perfect system – our body. Blind Max making his rounds in his wheelchair – slowly.

The psychic lady gave my wife a poem when she left the nursing home.

GUESTS

Pain knocked upon my door and said
That she had come to stay,
And though I would not welcome her
But bade her go away,

She entered in. Like my own shade
And followed after me,
And from her stabbing, stinging sword
No moment was I free.

And then one day another knocked
Most gently at my door.
I cried, "No, Pain is living here,
There is not room for more."

And then I heard His tender voice,
"Tis I, be not afraid."
And from the day He entered in,
The difference it made!

For though He did not bid her leave,
(My strange, unwelcome guest,)
He taught me how to live with her.
Oh, I had never guessed

That we could dwell so sweetly here,
My Lord and Pain and I,
Within this fragile house of clay
While years slip slowly by!
                    Author Unknown

December 10th – Home at Last, Noon

Home coming, third crush of tears. Attempted normalcy. Favorite reruns. **Highway to Heaven**, girls in prison, separated from their children. More tears.

Ruth cooked meatloaf. She's a star in this story. Friendship is caring, sharing, love.

The hospital bed keeps us separated at night. But, the twists and turns to adjust to pain – "the disturbance will keep you awake," she insists. Home is enough for now. We are together, under the same roof.

Radio Report at Noon
Highway jammed
Crash out of lanes
Hollywood at Highland
Suspected D.U.I. cause of collision

December 11th – Welcome Home

Security blanket, a few dollars tucked away for you darling when I die. And death is easy in this world. Remember, a fixed income leaves no room for increase of income. Books like movies, fail. **Patch**. Understandably, the mail lady should have followed her son's home on the bus. Surprise! Instead, reality. Fiction pleases people. Reality scares people. D.U.I. death reality.

In reality criminals escape punishment. In fiction the criminal always pays for the crime. The good-guy, bad-guy character is popular – a gray character with a black streak. In the news everyday.

The nursing home is a private world. A community of strangers united by pain and hope.

Our street is cookie cutouts of the same house pattern, slight variations. A few flags flying above doorsteps. Flowers and grass. The pallid blue sky. Sunset, sunrise – reflections on window panes. Our daily scenery.

No more Word Power Bingo, Piano Music, Church Service, Breakfast-Lunch-Dinner. Shower, change bedding, therapy, free walk, pain. Home Sweet Home.

A mask covering the eyes of the moon. **Long Ranger** in the morning. Return to the mundane. Normalcy. **Murder She Wrote** before bedtime.

The hoarseness diminished in her voice. She's taking with Valeria, twin survivors.

Reliving the collision. Details recalled.

"It was like you're watching a t.v. show. Watching you, and the air bag deployed.

Felt like my arm fell off. The mental sensation, a numbing pain circulating throughout my body.

In the crash I never lost consciousness. It was like I didn't want to lose consciousness. I watched you, Valeria. Your eyes closed, blood seeping from your lips. The first impact, shaking roughly."

The conversation continued. Careful review of the cause and extent of the injury. The mental state of recovery.

"We don't need to push sooner than we're ready."

"The car rushing toward us…"

The crash! The quick emergency response, cutting her loose.

The officer on scene interviewing the d.d. The statement by three passengers in the d.d. car experienced zero recall of the duel collisions. Sleeping was the explanation provided.

The officer at the scene of the collision, after addressing the driver, absolutely determined his condition of intoxication. The officer description and diagram exhibit the out of control drunk driver and the horrific results. My poor wife, battered and broken, very nearly killed.

Clothes cut away. Braces applied. Needles, pain relief, needles, blood transfusion, needles, I.V. medicine.

Our cars are mini-bombs. (A gas tank with mesh to prevent explosion is in production – too expensive to justify inclusion in auto safety.) Filled with gas – bolts, nuts, glass – shrapnel. 75 m.p.h. texting on the freeway – ring-a-bell. 75 m.p.h. D.U.I. college student – bombardier. Roadway bombs, sick people holding the detonator. In a hurry! 75 m.p.h. 80 m.p.h. 85 m.p.h. Destination unknown.

Zero tolerance D.U.I. M.A.D.D. College student? Anarchist? Senator?

College student?
Diverse nationality?   d.d. PLUS
Crowded jails
Holiday season

Testimony
Evidence   d.d. NEGITIVE
M.A.D.D.
Victims
Construction Zone

Questions of discussion. Does a judge hear testimony from victims? Does the judge hear about the people hit? The t.v. shows use lie detectors. How does the judge access the years of pain recovery? Lost of future years of life because of the d.d. collision damage to a normal body.

Can the average citizen figure out modern law? Plea agreement, no trial, justice served. A child's lose of finger control, future artist – absurd. A normal child with ordinary skill. Collusion will determine the worth of the child's injury. Do older people have arms of less value? Are there exceptions – surgeon, pianist, dart champion?

Picture a stranger walking in the park. Shoots eight bullets. A couple duck and hurt their backs. Four young people on the grass asleep, missed. One older woman grazed in the neck. Second older woman severely wounded. Three blood transfusions. Surgical implants. Braces. Pain pills. Pain.

No intent. Take his gun away. Send him back to college. Back to work and family. No one was killed. Stupid impulse of youth? Grave mistake of judgment? Alcoholic impairment? No pills! No drugs! Judge, this young man deserves another change.

Radio Traffic Sig-Alert
Crash on the 91
West before Adams
Semi – four cars
One fatality
D.U.I. suspected

December 12th

In the nursing home, a person is wheeled into a large shower stall, the nurse can walk around the person to assist the wash. Slightly more difficult in a standard bathtub. The support chair fits snug. The plastic laundry bucket provides a foot rest. To prevent knee bending with the brace off, a plastic coffee can cut open and wrapped over the knee, secured with duck tape. Lifting the braced leg into the tub was perilous. A t.v. commercial demonstration – the wrong way to bath an injury victim.

Phone Call – Sister.

"Can't lift my arm. I can move at the elbow and wrist. My fingers are fine. No chance of playing the violin. The therapist lifts my arm. Time and pain."

Her face, new lines – stress, pain, worry. Work for the golden years of retirement. You still share the road with the insane.

Car Chase #39. T.v. prime time. Ows and Ahs at intersections. Wow and woes, freeway acceleration. A time bomb ticking. The insane mind counting down.

December 13th

Clean-up the mess before the therapist arrives in the morning.

Moans consistent with movement. Like tennis players expulsion of breath. The tense discharge of stress. A reaction to pain. The sob, the grunt, the groan. New sounds in the home.

Sprinkles tonight.

Accident rate on Southern California freeways triples when rain falls. A slight precipitation on top of old oil stains produces slick roads. And speed limits rarely diminish in weather conditions considered superficial to Californians. Fog is the exception – sometimes.

Home therapy begins. Darwin, her visiting therapist, will provide the necessary steps to guide my wife to regain upper arm mobility. The knee pain, slow recovery. Ribs, slow recovery.

The healing capacity of our body is astonishing. However the speed is diminished by age.

Faith is a source of healing power.

Drugs to diminish pain alter a person's perception and character. Alcohol demonstrates the well established results of consumption altering the mental and physical state of a person's existence.

Radio Traffic Update
Crash in West L.A. on the 405
Traffic jammed before Forest Lawn
Drunk driver arrested

Ahhhhhh… Pain!

A left-handed pitcher, titanium plate attached with eight screws. Imagine a youth of eighteen, the wounded arm, mangled, crushed. Reconstructive surgery, ten inch incision, plate and screws. Stapled flesh – 44 stables.

Dear Lord,

The sky is clear. Stars bright. Thank You for the peaceful night. Thank You for a new day in our lives. Bless our loved ones and the people our lives touch here and hereafter, amen-Jesus- Jesus-amen.

December 14th

Enjoyed lasagna dinner with our dear friend, Ruth. We walked to her home down the street. My wife's lifelong friend. Superb cook.

Our daughter with grandparents visiting from Temecula. The great-grand child at the Disneyland parade.

Friends sharing a feast.

Check with the doctor, paper work. Write down questions. Degree of lose of arm strength? Family consultation. Lawyer?

Tomorrow, therapist – Darwin. Excellent therapist. Patience and guidance, a caring young man. Great conversationalist. A wife, child. Wonderful man. We are fortunate to have his help.

Conservatively $200,000 is spent on medical cost, before my wife is out of the nursing home.

Bail money, lawyer money, new car money. The cost generated by the teen driving drunk after an all night party. Stopped at Denny's. Brandy, Courvoisier, Rum in the coffee? The adult world. Rose colored glasses. A conceit. That reality does not apply. I am clear. Straight ahead. The car is power. Damn!

December 15th – Restriction on Life.
Phone Conversation – Valeria
"Apprehension driving home. The park flashing past. Cars everywhere. Overwhelming."

Note: Railing. Mobile chair. Bath.

My wife loves to shop. The children want her to visit the mall. They suggested rolling out the great grandma's old heavy wheelchair to shop over the holiday sales. Her foot extended is a problem. She vetoed the idea.

God Bless the children. Denial/Disbelief. The season of cheer. Her leg stuck out, her arm jolted on hard rubber wheels. Not impossible. But, best to side with caution. The nursing home is crowded this time of year.

Denial, disbelief. Most people cannot imagine their shoulder bashed by a bomb, the flesh deeply penetrated by a chunk of shrapnel. Same condition for my wife. Shoulder smashed, only the steel is inserted through a ten inch cut. Healing time, same. Pain time same. Pain intensity, same. Scar, same.

While talking on the phone, she shifted her weight, the chair legs slipped. She almost fell from the chair. One fall. Hip injury. Back to the nursing home. Extreme care is the guiding rule. No wheelchair in the shopping mall. Not this year.

In the afternoon she walked to the corner with her sister and grand-nephew – a soccer star. God does not spare children in car crashes. The wickedness of injury.

One car collision and one robbery – every American's statistical probability. The debilitating influence from drugs compounds the possibility of inflicting additional harm to the body. Maintaining arm immobility; leg locked at the knee – difficult adjustment required to recovery exercise and functional operations.

Her courage and perseverance is strong. My love. A walk on the pier. Next month? Next year?

Radio Traffic Sig-Alert
Traffic Crash in Long Beach
405 near Cherry
D.U.I. Curse

December 16th – Monday.
Visit from Valeria – new car. They are alive.
Doctor visit tomorrow X-Ray – knee surgery, preparation for surgery.

My wife swore today. An explicative directed at the one she loves. Drugs produce character change. Pain alters mood.

A comment in the car after the doctor visit. "Turn here, not there." Never allow the back seat driver to direct. You control the car, completely.

I neglected to help her into the car. She was too quick. One mistake, one fall. We are older. Weaker. Bones brittle.

Added stress. Added worry. Only a few days from the nursing home. The splint stays in place for a month – night and day. The arm remains motionless. Rush to return to normalcy. Damn!

The helplessness, the tiredness, the pills, pain, frailty, frilliness.

Venus bright! Monday night!

I remember the old couple, neighbors, died weeks apart. Occasional screams and oaths – obvious disagreement. They made me realize love can be temperamental at times. They mellowed with age.

My wife and I know what not to talk about. The list grows with the years passing.

Sexually, not able to do what is expected causes stress.

Radio Traffic Update
Crash earlier
Now on the shoulder
Injury crash, near Lakewood
D.U.I. arrest

********** ********** ********** **********

XII

X-ray

D.U.I. Victim… Surgeon statement,
"arm loss of function, pain."

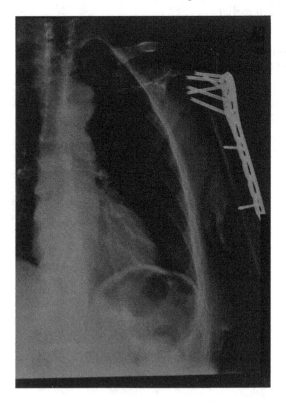

********** ********** ********** **********

XIII

Diary – Home Rehab

December 17th – No Response Ever.

Four healthy young men escape the double collision without a bruise. Two victims hospitalized. One injury, life threatening. Three I.V. transfusions of blood. Fractured ribs, severe bruising, leg immobilized, bone chips in knee, spine chips, arm cut open, 44 staples, plate and screws inserted. Four healthy men, unable to lift a pen to wish the older lady a thumbs-up.

Inappropriate, in a world of callous acceptance, rejection of accountability. The admission of guilt, avoidable. Anonymity maintained. The rights of the drunk driver must be protected.

No get-well card from Progress, Multi-State or Infinite. What passenger? Injury? Prove it!

December 17th – Night

Strap your arm to your side. Tape a tin can over your knee. Have a pleasant day. No driving or clapping or kicking field goals.

Multiply the handicap. Friend, neighbor, relative – highway victims on wheelchairs and crutches. My wife is lucky. Lucky to be alive. I am grateful.

People look at life through a bubble into reality. A thin transparent bubble, the thin line separating the infinite. Bubble burst, reality destroyed.

Inevitability…

Predestination…

Fate…

Never throw rocks at glass windows. Silly, what does a mind think, age eighteen, catapulted into the world where presidents are assassinated, drunk driving is a crime. D.U.I. collision victims last year – thousands and… My wife! Eight possible John and Jane Does.

Insurance companies officially discontinue claims. Agencies don't want to be connected to D.U.I. victims. Step away. 1, 2, 3. Not our problem. A criminal matter. The driver violated our trust. Complex. Legal.

Headline
Body discovered on the 5 freeway
Mystery

Fights, changing the will, money, drugs amplify emotion. Damn!

Shotgun blast at a college student party. What is happening in America, today?

Drugs. Booze. Violence. Guns.

Multiple personalities. Multiple combinations. Mix, mingle, maul. Text – Love!

Depression. Sleeping long hours.

Surgeon visit tomorrow. Question, crash victim psychiatric council. Victim and loved ones. Degree of motion loss? Degree of muscle lose? Degree of pain? Mental stability?

December 18th

Thankful my wife and Valeria survived the collision. Thankful no one was killed. The shock and damage. Realization, the holidays increase highway collisions. The extent of the pain. Christmas crazies.

The tweet – 75 mph – I love you. Innocent. Age 16. Deceased at the scene. Highway fatality.

The news distressing. T.v. show, hit and run recreation – realistic. My wife shaken by the sudden scene in a sea of calm. Shock impact, a writer's tool.

Lame excuse for inflicting violence – tweeting.

Denial of human limitations particular to operating two thousand pounds of machinery at 75 m.p.h. Simple. Point the wheels, press the gas pedal.

Valeria refuses to drive on the freeway. Her driving competence is superior. Of course, there is no driving defense against a drunk driver.

Our neighbor, Dean, said my wife looked like a Chemo-patient. Lose of weight and chalky complexion. The negativity of any remark relevant to her health. I keep silent.

Fight! I'm old looking.

No, no.

Pictures, forget it.

Perhaps the drugs make you feel smarter than normal people. Fight!

Ice cream is not…

Fight. Leave.

The beginning of the end.

If money were laughter, we'd all be clowns.

The newest crash claimed two lives – celebrities. Race car driver and actor, early 40's. $500,000 vehicle, suspected racing, excessive speed, smashed into a pole – disintegration and fire. (Ten million dollar settlement to heir.)

Easy to die a fool. Diana forgot to buckle her seat belt. We are all invincible.

We value the reckless rebel. James Dean – excessive speed. A hero. Take a dare – chicken.

$500,000 junk pile. Flowers on the sidewalk. Midnight race track. 7th street.

December 19th

Visit to the surgeon. Removal of leg brace.

The parking garage. "Turn around!" Screaming. Waiting for cars to pass. Screaming. "Turning around!" Invectives. Pain.

I'm convinced the drugs cause my wife's volatile outbursts. Calm composure is shattered by a curse. "You dummy. Do it wrong. Can't you see? Stupid!"

Not the same relationship since the d.d. established a macho image, survivor of a freeway mash.

God Bless us, dear Lord. Help guide us through the pain and confusion. Help heal the wounds. Amen-Jesus-Jesus-amen.

The weather has turned cold. Old bones ache. God Bless the nursing home.

December 20th

"Leave me alone." The morning greeting. A drug stupor. "I'm cold." Heater on the fritz. Next pay day. "Alone."

Radio Traffic
Woodland Hills
101 South Bend
Topanga Canyon
Ladder in left lane

What is left to say? My wife home safe. Perpetrator caught.

Necessary change, a box under her blanket to keep pressure off her knee.

My wife is several years older than my age. Men usually die younger than women. Since the collision her life expectance dropped. Pain kills.

I sleep more. Money problems. Knee patch, pills, heating blanket for hospital bed. My mom's final inheritance money slips away. Mom died three years ago. The house was sold and the siblings enjoyed the money – money equals fun, happiness – security. Lack of money equals sadness – anxiety.

I've always been fortunate – working. My wife worked. The problem is financial uncertainty. We live in an irresponsibly manipulated economy, government tomfoolery. We now live on a fixed income. Now, medical inflation. Plus, credit cards max.

Common, lower middle class people – welcome – upper lower class. The numbers never lie. A mortgage is the next logical step to consolidate bills and return to a plus account – borrowed money, the children will receive less inheritance. They'll understand. Growing old can be expensive.

A faulty step can knock you flat. Whistle shrill. "Honey, the remote fell on the floor. I can't reach."

Time to return to my wife. She needs me. End of diary entry.

Looking forward to the New Year.

December 20th – Night Pain.
Bitterness… The drudgery of rehab.

What we use every movement without motion or lifting capacity. Each step cautious – fear of knee pain.

People that have faced physical stress from injury know. A small pain can trouble the strongest man. A massive pain born by the weakest woman. Regardless of degree, pain conquers. Pain controls. Pain kills the will to breath. What would the psychic lady say? *Pray for calm!*

The heater is broken, the temperature dropping – credit card Christmas. My sweetheart in pain. The washer leaks. Car broke down.

My friend, Lee, broke three ribs in a motorcycle crash. The pain, excruciating. My wife has rib and spine damage. He was young when injured.

My wife complains of shoulder pain. She whimpers pathetically. Torture to my heart. Time! Time! Time! Pain! Pain! Pain! A plate the size of a twisted beer can – screws for insertion. Cut flesh, forty staples. Pain…

Impact force to shoulder – 60 m.p.h. slam into resistant surface. Nearly hurricane speed. Highway injury. Catastrophic pain.

My wife is laughing, talking to her friend, Shirley, on the phone. Shirley survived cancer and pneumonia. Women suffer. Live longer. Courage.

I listened to my wife talk. "How does the body aura suffer a savage blow? The psychic lady knew the answer. Certainly she knew my condition. No warning. Worry for no reason. Aura intact, color slightly streaked with denser hues to concentrate healing force."

Strange words. Strange world, the healing mind searching for answers, reassurance, fabrication.

December 21st

Chicken, brown rice, zucchini, five cheese lasagna, meatloaf, potatoes. American cuisine. Home cooking from packaged frozen entries. Fresh salad – lettuce tomato, cucumber, carrots.

Cold-Cold-Cold. California shudders – low fifties. Wayne and Gale visited in the afternoon. A brief stop. He prayed for our health. A strong man, in late sixties. Kind and dedicated. People helping people are a blessing.

Peaceful night. Talking to the lamppost at midnight.

You growl like a basset hound, with a bite like a Chihuahua.

December 22nd

My wife looks at the pictures on her phone. The day the surgeon allowed her to remove her leg brace. The railroad track of band-aids climbs her shoulder. Each breath rib pain distorts her smile.

The house is cold. Car problem – the clutch – emptied the checking account. My wife's salary – merry Christmas money – vanished. All couples complain of finances.

We received a check from insurance company – $3000 settlement money for medical costs before medical costs are completed. Collision date wrong. Make sense! Lawyer directed us to return check.

Six weeks, waiting for a jail sentence, consulting with lawyer – the adult world. D.U.I. teen free, home without a care in the world. The public lawyer defends the drunk driver. Life continues. Waiting. No physical pain. No financial worry. Insurance covers costs. Initial problem, stay out of jail. Easy! Mercy of the court. No pain. Mental distress. No pain. No jail. Waiting…

Condition of penalty for drunk teen driver recklessly initiating the extinction of eight humans?

One thing. Wrong place – D.U.I. – wrong time.

Accelerated away from 1st car collision and accelerated away from 2nd car collision. Smoke obscuring vision – Construction Zone – darkness – accelerating D.U.I. maniac.

Hang him for his bad poetry.

Hang him for his bad lies.

December 23rd

Crying in her bedroom. Cold and sad. The Christmas songs, message of peace, good-will, joy. How close to her last Christmas? Holiday cheer – D.U.I. Celebration with pain. Alive! Alive! Alive!

Amazing how words can reflect a moment's intensity. A sigh, heartbeat, quiver – real mental images – cellular transference like in a dream. Teeth grinding, fear, relief. Realization – blindness. The siren's blue spin. Pain!

My darling bride. Indisposed. All messed up! Beaten down! Knee pain, belly pain, back pain, shoulder pain, arm pain, pain, pain, pain. Enough energy generated from nursing home pain to power a widget factory.

A new slice of moon, a hummock in the sky. Restful, clouds passing by, creeping softly. Venus, dazzlingly bright.

Time to say a prayer for our nursing home friends. We will remember you, always. Our prayers, always. God Bless!

A sweep of clouds cover the northern sky, advancing. Rain clouds for thirsty California. Trouble for the middle bunk in room 14A. Trouble for the home without heat. Trouble for the old ache and pain. Trouble we need. Quarter inch rain. Wow!

We complain about a meaningless event – cold day. Never satisfied. Life owes me. What's in it for me? Capitalistic normalcy.

My wife has a new batch of drugs. The pain is dulled – in check. She will sleep, peacefully.

So many highway victims struggle every day to repair the injury, usually avoidable injury. We are only human. A mistake can happen. I can text and drive – multi-task. D.U.I. – one drink! In a hurry? Prescription medicine.

T.V. screen with internet contact on the dashboard. What could possibly go wrong?.

December 24th

Rain today. Therapy canceled. Last night the pain caused a vomit seizure. New pill prescription. The body discharges foods unnaturally, a serious sign of illness. Scary.

I suppose it is natural to shift thought to anger toward the person responsible for the disturbing change to our lives.

A young man, healthy, quickly learning to make the system work to his advantage. A card shark stacking the deck. Leniency. No! No one was killed. A lifeline shortened. Forgivable.

Damn the d.d. soul and the devil that spawned the d.d. Damn every f…ing drunk on the road today and forever. Damn them to hell.

Norman Vincent Peal – **The Power of Positive Thinking.** Do not allow the invasion of negative thought into the mind and heart and soul. Faith! Forgive!

The vulnerability of age. Miscalculated expense. Financial abuse. Medical catastrophe. Illness. Age!

The perfect picture. Age with health, die in sleep. My neighbor, robust, healthy, age 90 – diabetic – leg amputation to preserve his life. He lasted six months. The torture! The pain!

The vulnerability of age.

I thought age lead to greater respect. No! Age leads to weakness. Take advantage of the old – easy! Fraud and deceit. The old are weak.

Depend on no one but yourself. Question everything. Keep an open mind. Pray.

December 25th – Merry Christmas!

Christmas calls to family, friends. No travel this year.

Sparks from sunset; whisper from the surf. A walk along Sunset Beach. The Old King's Bridge; El Camino Real swept by the tides. My mother-in-law painted the seascapes, artist trying to capture a personal treasure from God's masterpiece.

Bath: choreograph every move. Rehearse every step. Caution!

Family pictures. Christmas songs, holiday cheer make the burden of pain easier to bear. Still hurts! Every drop of one degree of pain is a victory. Sunny day, kind word, Christmas – one, two, three... **Joy-to-the-World**... four, five... **Peace on Earth**...

Titanium screws take time to seal with bone and flesh. Like titanium teeth implants, the process is slow for complete amalgamation of the metal inside the body. Resistance, rejection possible. Her spirits are high. Six... **Jingle Bells.**

Remember, the wrong move erases the pain degree numbers dropped and quite possible will add a degree of pain. Careful, choreograph every move before engaging movement. Visualize the steps necessary to complete a task or physical adjustment. Slow step by step by step…

Baby steps. Mimic Madalyn Rose.

Our hearts are blessed, this Christmas and every Christmas.

December 26th

Skip bail. Travel back to his grandfather's country, live with relatives, begin a new life. Did the d.d. celebrate Christmas? Happy eggnog!

All was well today. No verbal flare-up. Perhaps a warmer day, no cold rain. The heater will be fixed this week. Borrowed money for the repair. The thousand dollar clutch repair depleted the checking account. Credit card bills cancel savings. Add the new challenge of meeting the medical costs. Damn!

Friends will add a rail to the porch. Shorter steps cemented in place. Someday soon.

We are lucky. We make ends meet. So many poor people, homeless sharing Christmas in the streets.

I always thought American's elected representatives capable of maintaining effective government. Our debt makes fools of generations of elected officials, obviously the majority incapable of responsible economics.

Social experiment the guiding principle of modern government. The greatest country on earth, denied prosperity. Incredible.

The nursing homes in California. Inspected once every five years. Imagine our jails receiving incompetent service. Someone might complain.

Radio Traffic Alert
Car flipped
Nightmare jam 210
Use alternate route
Western Highway clear

Back to normal. My wife and Ruth shopping for after Christmas goodies. A pair of ankle weights added to this year's Christmas list.

The granddaughter visited. New drivers license – no insurance. No money! Innocence! Ignorance! Perhaps she is insured under the owner of the vehicles policy. Think positive.

Medical coverage is guaranteed by government law. Why worry. Besides, odds are fifty-fifty the other driver in a collision has insurance.

Everyone forgets to signal when changing lanes on a freeway. Everyone breaks laws. Do I need insurance for the few hours driven each week? A trip to the corner market. Driving my sister to school.

A truck driver, hauling cross country, needs insurance. Small time drivers – optional. College students exempt! Think of the world.

What is the worst that can happen – D.U.I. Recently a basketball player, D.U.I. conviction – three years probation. M.A.D.D. The message: ignore blood alcohol level in the big boys. College students, too! Congressmen? Probation!

December 27th – A Walk on the Beach.

I must return to my primary mission as an educator and lexicographer. Make the dictionary publishers underline English/Spanish cognates/cognadoes in future dictionaries. Simple, effective method of assisting future Americans to comprehend our forefather's languages when the constitution was written – English and Spanish. Realize the number of English/Spanish cognates in our Constitution is extensive.

My beach poem effort is dark. I was thinking of Poe and his poem, **Lenore**.

Beach Poem #309

No footsteps on the sand
No clouds in the sky
No merriment
No laughter
The winds hollow cry.

Dark seascape
Cold shadows
Hostile waves
Night storm
Mudslides/debris
Eminent causality

Friday
P.C.H.
Fatality
The spirits of the dead
Haunting the shore
Screaming

December 28th

Dearest, define pain and suffering. List for our lawyer.

1... Intolerable pain – arm, back & knee cap.
2... Lashing out at my husband – frustrated.
3... Feeling like an invalid for the 'little' things I cannot do.
4... My body has lost so much weight that makes me look gaunt, skin & bones – WEAK.
5... People say I look like I have lost too much weight – 'fatten up.'
6... OMG – go outside, go to store – may look like I am OK but injuries are internal – the pain is there instantly. Orders from surgeon, no pressure on left arm. Next appointment with him in January. Some motion is OK.
7... I secretly cry.

The heater pilot light went out. I'm to blame. My wife insists looking at the pilot. We did not realize the task of returning to her feet. We wedge her back against a chair, I lift her back up, place a foot stool under her butt; she slides upward until both feet touch ground. Frustrating! More negative sparks.

She is weak, feels chills, quick tempered. The forces of evil built with pain. Waves of pain. The soul confused by the relentless onslaught. Question? Seek a new temple? Time to move along? Too much pain! Mixed message; mental strain.

Ambushed at dawn by a demon. The power of the devil in the hands of a drunk teenager. Damn! Damn!

Seventy degrees predicted for tomorrow. Bright outlook. Positive thinking. She is recovering. Each day stronger.

The devil cannot win.

Half moon center of the sky.
Wait!
Pray…

December 29th
Mental Imagery
A gift, petals blooming.
White roses, silver bow.

A magic bracelet.
Glitter paint, pink and gold.

Smiling Madalyn Rose.
Balloons and Hats.

Candles on her birthday cake.
Angel and Cross.

Radio Report.
Crash on Highway 22
Blocking two lanes.
Fatality.

Highway, ant columns, vehicles bump, limbs break, flesh tears. Pain and suffering.

I cry secretly. Ashamed to admit the weakness to pain. The drain of energy – pain. Pain and suffering defined. A blurred message. Individual pain tolerance and extent of injury – subjective balance impossible to measure.

Grandmother has a sore back from hoeing the garden.

Sharp, jabbing pain, like a splinter under the skin. A splinter of pain charged with a jolt of hot energy, shocking pain. Work pain will go away, not the same as injury pain.

Crash victims injured survive. Why me? Pain inflicted by a freeway drunk is unfair. Pain beyond work pain and age pain. A wicked, wicked pain. Electric pain!

December 30th – Morning Pain.

"Today I woke-up again in so much pain… my back, arm and knee. The same pain that will get better but it is taking so much time. What a slow healing process. On this blessed day, is my son's birthday. We called him and sang happy birthday. What if I could not?"

Loss of normal activity. List for our lawyer.

1... Missing some fun.
2... Dinner on the patio, our favorite restaurant, a view of the sea.
3... Walks on the pier. The rough planks vibrating from crashing waves.
4... Driving to the mountain resorts. Palm Springs. Laughlin, Nevada.
5... Lawn bowling in our back yard.
6... Missing retirement.

Start a charity for nursing homes. Distribute money for improvement of comforts – garden beauty – t.v. reception – poster boards for family display. Art – painting and sculpture. Fake flowers. Puzzles, magazines, books. Nothing fancy or extreme. No bonus pay or treatment reimbursement. Donut cushions and ice packs. Comfort, warm socks with skid preventers.

Newspaper story: the son shot his mother suffering from dementia. Then he went to the nursing home and shot his sister in the head. She was in a coma for five years after a D.U.I. car crash. He went to the patio and waited for the police.

A day without pain!

December 31st

Six weeks, no lights around the porch, Santa, sled and rain-deer missing. A snowman perched by the door – the sole Christmas attraction.

A tree on the kitchen table this year – two feet tall. The hospital bed takes up Christmas tree space.

A gingerbread house on the lamp table. The manger scene on the mantel of the electric fire place.

Last years elves and giant candy canes still wrapped and stored away.

This Christmas filled with joy. Amen-Jesus-Jesus-Amen. Life the precious gift.

January 1st

The final statement of fact. The pain will be there – at different degrees – for her lifetime. Diminished by treatment and drugs, the pain will always be part of her life. The positive twist, her survival. My greatest reward, ever.

Today a woman, 64, killed in a seven-car crash caused by a speeding driver. The speeder walked away from the collision into a store, bought a six pack of beer, sat on the curb drinking when approached by police. Strange, perhaps a mental breakdown.

People rushed to aid the injured in the crashed vehicles. Crash! Crash! Crash! A woman stopped at a red light. Pronounced dead at the scene of the collision.

Christmas Crazies dramatically increase daily Crash Ratio on American highways.

I see an unsure future of major concern and consequence. An uncertain year projected. The unexpected. A new baby unpredictable future.

God Bless my wife. The pain will subside, disappear. Hopefully! God Bless the Nursing Home. God Bless the New Year.

January 2nd – Sunday Night.

The warmer day is a blessing for aches. The cold intensifies pain. The blood is drawn inward, away from joints. Surface tissue cools, muscles contract, nerves strain – pain. The warmth relaxes the body, blood flows naturally, soothing nerves. One degree less pain.

January 3rd – Judy

My wife has lost interest in television entertainment. She retries to bed early. She says the violence disturbs her. You can see a dozen car crash scenes, even commercial dummy impact – channel surf and the numbers multiply.

Do people mimic the crazy car scenes on t.v. and movies? Do teens mimic race car drivers? Fast and furious race?

We visited Judy this morning at the nursing home. We talked on the patio – eighty degrees in Long Beach. Her weight is down, bacterial infection controlled, her knee strength slowly returning. Faith and exercise. Strong heart. Patience. Prayer!

The slightest comfort makes a difference. My wife explained how her pain was eased in the hospital by pillows propped around her body, holding her softly. Another degree less of pain.

The lightest comfort makes a difference. A kind word.

The puzzle book is Judy's distraction. **Inspirational Word Find**, **Jumbo Word Find** and **Movie Word Find**. We always bring Judy a new book when we visit.

Today: **Chicken Soup for the Soul Word Find**.

January 3rd – Night.

"Honey, how's the pain?"

"Oh. It's there."

Resignation... who cares... why complain... apathy... pain with a capital P, capital A, capital I, capital N.

Endurance.

Difficult to continue the diary. Depressive reflection, repetitive pain imagery.

Teeter-totter ride. Sometimes up, sometimes down.

My heart leaps with joy, my bride is safe. She is home. We are together.

The pain, drugs, incapacitation, restriction, finality, impedance, moans in the night – negative thought and depressive emotion.

I'm going to work on the sea poems. Sunshine beaches, the power of thundering waves, playful dolphin. A walk on the pier. Next week. Soon.

January 4th

Hospital bed returned. Home therapy suspended. Drug dose reduced. Pain continues. The support has been tremendous. Time to move forward together, with help from friends and family, surgeon and God.

Back surgery rescheduled. Surgery on knee three weeks to wait. Back surgery postponed until weight stabilized. Worry, worry, worry. Fear!

January 5th
Radio Sig-Alert
Crash involves a big rig
All lanes are down
D.U.I. driver arrested

Shopping with sister. My wife carries a cane. She explained the specialized standing cane adjustments. Pain in back along nerve – sacroiliac. Sharp, jabbing pain. Damn!

Clear and cool evening. Tomorrow seventy degrees.

January 6th
Stomach cramps, bowel malady. Neck and shoulder persistent pain; knee-hip-back pain. First week of New Year – pale, tired, settled in bed – six o'clock. Drug reaction evident, languid. Chills!

Last year her normal vivaciousness, light of the party, helping to spotlight Jesus.

An Angel wing cushioned her body the terrible morning the car rammed the concrete wall. The other wing cushioned her friend. Our hearts are blessed by God's love.

The psychic lady told my wife an Angel feather granted a wish. I wish for my wife to be healthy.

Night. The roar of voices. The recording in our mind. Laughter, howling wind, moans and groans. The buzz of the infinite stars. The moon, rumble and roll.

After-hour at the Continental Lounge. Pink, bubbly champagne. This year return to the Queen Mary. Memories of the passionate night, our embrace, kiss at midnight, New Year's Eve. Maybe next year.

Helicopter circling Vons parking lot. White light flashing. Tomorrow morning headline.

January 7th

Six people walk away. The d.d. walks away. Only my wife damaged, fate-line altered. No more fishing fun. Unwanted pain. She is not alone. Each year thousands of names are added to the list of highway victims – dead and wounded. A cruel price to pay. Forgotten, left to their own resources to survive.

All day in bed. Complain of pain. Cries. Complaining of complaining. A sad confusion. Pain for complaining. Damn!

She adapts. She takes a pill for pain. She sleeps more. Mobility increases back pain. Cries, moans, whimpers. Damn!

January 8th

Can't quite get the tilted picture on the wall to stand straight. A slight tremble in the hands, a little more gray. Minor change. Helping my bride recover is a full time job.

Vigilance, compassion, hide-the-worry, smile.

Words become reminders of pain like blood drops on the page.

Gloom and doom. A fit of rage to see her suffer. Realize the savagery of highway collisions. Needless destruction.

Abhorrent.

86% increase in car crash on holiday time.

Does the d.d. keep a diary. Reveal thoughts of that morning before dawn. His suffering. Regret. Admission of guilt? Private thoughts. A coward's silence.

January 9th

Freida Kahlo expressed pain in her paintings. A young women, a bus accident, a lifetime of pain – no children. Degree of tragedy. Women are strong. Hospital Bed painting. Fruit Basket painting. The detail.

A painting of a women. Pain in her eyes. A women in the orchard. Reaching for an apple. Right arm only. Curious the details come to mind individually and collectively. We all experience pain. The twist of an ankle, the cut of a knife. A splinter. Lost toy. Scolding. Burn.

Bigger pain, broken arm, broken heart, cramps. Big, bigger pain, the root canal, poison ivy, migraines, back ache. Biggest pain, any of the above sustained permanently, day-by-day, night-after-night.

Slow, slow increase in color tone, pale to pink. Weight, skin tightness, muscles need increased exercise.

Tomorrow, a lunch date with friends. And, a trip to the nursing home to visit with Judy. Judy is standing.

January 9th – Night.

My poor darling, the months of pain, a long toothache. She looks like a child expecting punishment. The questioning look. For what reason? The tears. Pain!

The night is cool, the Big Dipper hanging above the horizon. Holiday celebrations ended. Office party! Champagne lunch! Free beer at the bar! Yahoo!

A d.d. drove into a house and killed a man in bed. Drink and speeding. Rush! Rush! Rush!

Prohibition failed. Common sense failed. Will justice fail? Consequence and accountability.

The d.d. free to drink alcohol the day released from jail.

January 10th

Morphine Sulfur – 15 MG table – one tablet twice a day

Hydrocodone – Acetaminophen 5-325 – 1 tablet 3 times a day for severe pain

Aleveeee…

January 11th

Minimal change to report.

New trial date for d.d. Second postponement.

Repetition of information ingrained in the brain, like a record groove deeper and deeper. Repetition of a sensation, the record over and over, the grove deeper and deeper. The message of pain, the record never stops playing.

The mistake remembered and repeated in memory, the groove deeper and deeper. Punishment reinforced by the whip and chain.

Positive memory zapped by electric shock. The canvas wrinkled and torn. Health in delicate balance. New Year plans? Go Forward Bravely.

Visit with Judy yesterday was fun. Tired tonight. Friends call. We'll watch the news, sports. I was born in Buffalo, New York. Bills! My wife is a California girl. Real blonde. Smart. 49er fan!

Wake-up one morning with severe bursitis in the shoulder region. Nerve up the neck, down the spin screaming pain. The back pain. Knee pain. Arthritic seeds planted deep. Damn!

Grateful for her healing day-by-day. Grateful for the warm weather. Friendship and Love.

We need more laughter. A source of healing power. Cartoons with car crashes, common? **Mad, Mad, Mad World**. Collapsing piano is funny. Commercials. A collapsing piano in a commercial. The *k* sound is funny. Coffee! Kangaroo! Kristin!

January 12th – Night.

A quiet day, reading. My wife watched a romantic drama in black and white – Kurt Douglas. Rugged looks, handsome.

I hold her shoulder like holding a dove. Gentle massage. The flesh is shrunken, muscles weak, movement painful.

Curious, to write the same information everyday in a different form of description, word variation. Pain and Beauty.

Eighteen orchid blossoms on a stem in the garden, the plant from my mother-in-law. God rest her gentle soul. White, with gold and red flakes. Every flower, artful perfection.

My wife reminds me, the trash goes out.

"I Love you Honey."

"I Love you Sweetie."

Tomorrow she shops with Ruth. The tedium of life continues. With pain and drugs to weaken the heart. Her lassitude scares me.

Laughter! Ha! Ha! Ha!

January 13th

Permanence that is an illusionary tract between life and death.

January 14th

Sent Orange County Probation Department questionnaire about d.d. No response.

My wife is old school, home chores a woman's work. We share after I insisted vacuum and laundry are tough tasks.

My wife can't lift, push, or carry. No weight over five pounds. No scrubbing, vacuuming, laundry limited, cooking restricted. God Bless her. Dressing is a difficult task. One arm, back aching. Slow and easy. No sharp movement. Knee bend, ouch. Long sleeve thermo for warmth.

January 15th

New letter for our lawyer. Justice for D.U.I. crime – undetermined. Civil Trial for reasonable restitution? Legal costs? Insurance responds? Questions for the expert.

The complexity of the legal system requires expert interpretation. Checkbook justice; the most zeros wins. D.U.I. crime? Probation? Justice? A D.U.I. jail or camp to break rocks and think – repent. Commit to a productive honest life. No more alcohol!

Can't buy back time. Money can't secure the future. Money can cheer-up the present. No amount of money can stop pain.

With government control of the insurance industry, all money is in question.

Advice of a friend. "Make the system work for you."

Public Defender. Insurance lawyer. Bail provided. Legal leniency. The system works for the D.U.I. criminal.

Clouds passing over; black cat crossing the yard.

The curse of pain.

A life-line shortened?

January 16th

Paper work, complete forms, collect information, respond before court date. A freeway bump-and-grind, spin-out, fender-bender. The true picture is a battle scene, twisted metal and one shattered body. And, the calm recovery of the d.d. and his passengers. Carnage by cowards. Run and hide, lying cowards.

And the lesson learned. No big deal. Cuts and bruises. No one is going to jail. Forgive and Forget. The pain will go away. They are old. They die, soon.

No super volcano. No asteroid strike. Human continues to bump into human. The magnitude of individual identity is the gift of God. Motorist expendable.

Appearance is deceptive. Internal complications, invisible injury. Movement without pain is impossible. No sleeping on left side. Her knee is not right. Back aching. All symptoms undetectable by the eye. Dizziness. Chocking.

January 17th
1,400 hit-and-run reports in the L.A. area – one year. 1,400 highway victims denied justice. Now, the text-generation. What penalty for a collision caused by a texting driver on a freeway, fast lane – eighty miles per hour? Phone time never wrong. Smashing into two cars, pain and suffering evident. Reckless driving. No jail time. Insurance release, return of license.

Turn on the Internet Screen! No problem with reception even at 80 m.p.h.

Will our highway tragedies increase before the newest technology makes our highways safer? The human factor the greatest cause of disaster. Rarely do brakes fail, speed increase or decrease without the effort of the human foot. Tail-lights don't signal unless you flick the switch. You must put gas in the gas tank. Turn the key in the ignition. Search your mind for every step in driving procedure to reach the corner of the block. One, two, three four, five, six, seven, eight, nine…

January 18th – Super Bowl Invitation, Vegas.
Shopping with her sister a few hours, exhaustion. Loss of appetite, nausea, pain down back. Fear of surgery. The shoulder serious pain, the surgeon will explain on Monday.

Football games ending the season, who wins, who retires to ignominy? Our taste for the bruising sports has diminished. We are looking forward to baseball.

Looking forward to summer sunshine. Less pain. Peace.

Full Moon.

Fun canceled.

January 19th

Pick-up medical cost paper at nursing home. Visit Judy – orchid and word puzzle book. Beauty for the heart, exercise for the brain. A positive boost for the physical pain.

Surgeon report positive. Therapy continues. Pain will continue during therapy. Special diet for weight improvement prescribed.

Three months dedicated to the healing process. Two pounds down in weight in two days. Appetite weak, sad, sad, sad. Thousands of Americans suffer the same fate. Needless pain. Needless waste. Texting. D.U.I. Drugs. Speeding.

More sad news. A morning crash killed three – age 20, 18, 19. One survivor. Return from all night party. Fire. D.U.I.

Check your policy, watch for D.U.I. coverage guaranteed.

Your agent insured the driver, the law breaker. In good faith, the company accepted responsibility for the driver's credibility as a capable and honest individual, licensed to drive a vehicle. The insured driver reneged on the insurance agreement. The driver caused a collision while intoxicated. No effort to assist the victims was documented.

The medical condition of one victim continues to be impossible to predict. Is liability for costs the responsibility of the insurance company or the d.d.

Reimbursement of loss of average years of life by highway victims conditional to severity of collision and predicable lifespan.

Blab. Blab. Blab.
Fear, step by step, fear.

January 20th
Radio Traffic Tragedy
Crash on P.C.H.
Two intoxicated motorists.
Child passenger killed.
Sig-alert cleared.

Alcohol, a major contribution to our social development.

Defensive Driving. How to defend against a drunk driver in the dark exceeding 75 m.p.h. in a Construction Zone – blindsided collision. Impossible defense. Check-mate.

My anger continues to spill out every time I put a pen to paper.

The poetry book seems trivial compared to my wife's dilemma. I will continue with the sea poems. Her mom's pictures in print will cheer-her-up.

Food – exercise – muscle.

Feels like we took a few sudden steps up Jacob's Ladder. Still a ways to the top. God guide our steps.

January 21st
Her surgeon, young, optimistic – 6 months? 1 year? The end of pain, no guarantee. Therapy will hurt. Limitations unpredictable at present. Reevaluation date in three weeks. Weight gains first priority.

Knee, back condition evaluation incomplete.

One woman's pain, a sad reminder of another D.U.I. collision.

Hit-and-Run. Slap on the wrist. No insurance reimbursement for injury. No D.U.I. policy. Minimum coverage for teen motorists. Standard case.

Senior citizen victim. Common citizen. Civil War ancestry. Father: W.W.II veteran. No political fame. Postal clerk. Husband: School teacher. Retired.

Radio Traffic Alert
Crash in a Construction Zone
One mile south of Garden Grove
Spinning road, air bags explode

January 22nd
New washer arrives tomorrow – $800. Mini-loads for a long time in the old machine.

Many situations questionable. Medical condition questionable. Go forward bravely.

Hit-and-Run causality today. Three cars collided. Faulty driver fled scene with two passengers. Cowards!

January 23rd – Night
Full Moon – Big Dipper
Liability – Party Host?
Increased pain with therapy.

Giant Full Moon.
Write the provocative, captivating – page galloping pace. Common and repetitive. Wheelchairs spinning, after the amateur race car driver loses.

Faceless parade of people. No age, gender or race. Victims of road madness and rage.

We live in a delusional world. Year-by-year our mortality guaranteed. The innocent acceptance shattered by the unpredictable future – good or bad. Displacement of a common timeline by a d.d. Apathy/Acceptability.

Shopping with her sister. "A shame to have the pain." They enjoyed the visit.

The weakest link, moving too fast, step first, jump later.

Sent poems and dictionary to police officer, our hero.

Dictionary to help communication in our bilingual state. Poem collection for relaxation.

Alarm! Alarma! A twist fist signal.

Emergency information is essential to communicate correctly. Recognition of vocabulary identical in English and Spanish is important for police and citizen. Future generations will appreciate present improvement of recognizing the fraternal relationship of English and Spanish. 90% of the major words in this paragraph are English/ Spanish cognates/cognadoes.

English/Spanish Crossover Diccionario produced for California bi-lingual students.

January 24th

Legal term – malicious wounding… a scar?

The moon rising over the peak of the house, up above the palm trees, reaching for Venus racing into black.

My wife visited our great-grandchild. No lifting. Hugging heart to heart. Kisses. Joys of life.

Her car seat needs an airbag bubble.

January 25th

Watching the play-off football match-up replay on television. Sport news always replay the worst collisions on the gridiron. Knee injury – player carried off the field. My wife – grimace. She knows the pain. She knows the long recovery. Football heroes!

Papers need to be filed. Court date deadline draws near. Outcome unknown. Speculate zero alteration in d.d. lifeline. Driving privilege reinstated – insurance pays for car repair. Back to school. Hang with the crew. Party time. No problem. No pain! Old people damage, negligible.

January 26th – Back to Work.

Memory never lost, simply slowed down, crowded with age. Medical paper requested from hospital. Thirteen day wait by mail, no delivery and needed for court evidence. The court must be notified on a specific date. Failure to provide required information is victim's negligence.

My wife does not sleep well. Restriction of movement, pain. Excessive time in bed with too little sleep. Less drugs, more pain, less sleep. A pattern is evident.

Out patient therapy the next obstacle. The surgeon explained therapy would increase pain. Weight loss serious concern. Two more pounds lost this week. Dizziness.

Positive thought. Faith! The greatest suffering is behind her. The leg brace removed until knee surgery. She is mobile. Functional. Perhaps the sudden activity burns calories faster. The bright picture spotted with black.

Pain causes weariness. Energy loss, weight loss. Exercise equals more pain. Depression. Why try!

Aging naturally is tough enough without unwanted handicaps inflicted without reason.

The diary is dark, the texture of each page gloom. The positive story sides with youth. A foolish mistake. Won't happen ever again. Back to girlfriend and crew. Parental support. Legal rigmarole. A system to busy and to crowded to bother with another D.U.I. crime.

D.U.I. released three times, kills a motorcyclist, released after nine months in jail. True story!

Radio Traffic – Noon
Crash in South Gate
West 710
Suspected D.U.I. motorist

January 27th .

Physically pick-up important documents, no mail, no fax, no U.P.S. – face to face pick-up – good advice.

Argument about directions to pick-up hospital bill. Good advise – don't argue with spouse. Sorry is the most important word in a marriage.

Another drive to the U.C.I. hospital, court document to establish evidence of injury. $250,000 dollar injury with continuing medical expense, undetermined. Eight people in the collision – cost of injury multiplied. Wow! Death is cheaper.

Death is close. Death walks near hospitals, nursing homes, highways. Opening the door for death is easy – drink & drive.

The passage of time is swift, consumed by the recovery process.

Radio Traffic – Noon
Traffic jammed solid
Crash in South L.A. on the 110
No fatality

Tweet: no money, no fame. Common sense insistence: dictionary publishers underline English/Spanish cognates/ cognadoes in future dictionaries. Lexicographers agree, a good idea.

January 28th

d.d. diary

"Why did it happen to me?"

Random selection? Pitchfork from hell!

"Thank God the old bitch didn't die. I'm fucked. Death is bad news. Possible jail time. Gonna get her picture bouncing around. Complete recovery! The old bitch! Can't shake-down me. I'm not stupid. I know the score. Lawsuit. Hypocrite! Old bitch! Progress will defend my ass. For sure!"

Streak clouds tonight. Mystic blue at sunset. Warm! Excellent healing weather. Minnesota children: forty degrees below zero. Dangerous. Mother Nature fills the most graveyards.

Man killing man. Accidents. Devine force. Stupidity.

Grace and Mercy.

January 29th

Smart drivers carry uninsured motorist insurance for maximum dollars. Three drivers in D.U.I. collision carried the minimum insurance required by law. In the past checking the square for uninsured motorist meant full coverage. Big mistake! Times change. Rules change.

Carry the maximum possible of the uninsured motorist coverage.

Knowledge is only valuable before the need for protection. Evidently the d.d. coverage is limited. Insurance never pays an extra dime without legal justification. Additional coverage for 'high risk' motorists – unnecessary. Why protect normal motorist from 'high risk' teenage drivers or convicted drunk drivers? Facts often lie.

Financial restitution for injury resulting in restricted use of left arm is inconsequential in comparison to the grave highway injuries and highway death. Not a dollar for pain.

Criminal accountability – zero? Jail? Victim restitution?

January 30th
"Sharp pain in my arm."

Our great-grandchild, eight months, standing. Perfection.

Ma and Pa belong to a car club. Find a member to build a bubble baby car seat. A seat that releases air bags to cocoon the baby. A gift for Madalyn Rose.

January 31st
"I have not been happy since the collision."

I love to hear my wife laughing, her voice exciting. She will pause to listen, and inject an exclamation, a positive wow!

The tremor of pain in the voice you love, a new note, low note.

Our love life is strained. Karma Sutra for Impaired. We experiment. Carefully. The tangle of limbs, impossible.

The moon, a canoe rowing through clouds.

Twenty-six year old husband of the nurse in the doctor's office. He was killed – car smashed into a freeway wall. D.U.I. victim.

Radio: Traffic Sig-Alert
South Gate on the 710
Three car smash-up
D.U.I. arrest

February 1st
Holiday = 86% increase in accidents
Rain = triple number of accidents

D.U.I. = …… % increase in holiday accidents
Texting = …… % increase in holiday accidents

___

Total = Highway Motorcide

Clouds, rain showers. A sense of order. The jigsaw puzzle piece fitting perfectly. A complete picture. Acceptance of change dependent on need – coincidental circumstance.

The guarantee canceled.

Radio Traffic – Fatality.
Trip to the super store
Lady with a cell phone
Racing through the Construction Zone
Crashing into the wall

February 2nd

February 2nd
Serious problem with the palate fit of dentures. Weight loss obvious cause of dental destress. New clothes, new belts, new bras. New wardrobe, overnight. New body, label attached – fragile.

She was stripped of a layer of flesh, like stripping off a neoprene wetsuit. The rubbery layer gone. Wrinkled parchment, the crumbled newspaper page, 1940 – easily torn.

Blue eyes, intelligent, light spirited, wise.

Radio: Traffic Sig-Alert
Car wreck in the right lane.
Overturned motorcycle
One fatality
D.U.I. victim

Writer's Digest poetry contest. Time to enter again this year. Compulsive thoughts of collision, near death d.d. collision. Sad.

D.U.I. Victim Case #13NF20100

Construction Zone east exit Forest Lawn
18-inch tall reflectorized orange cones
new white lines, parallel, straight
uniform as the footsteps of a Saint

65 mph crash into the freeway stone wall
extended heartbeat between here and heaven
mirror with blood drops on cracked lips
face ashen, clammy; cold, pellucid stare

shriek of metal slashing concrete
sparks flash, airbag impact, whiplash
flesh stretching and tearing
bones chipped and cracked

electric spread of nightmare pain
taillight streaks whirling insane
2nd detonation, screeching rubber burns
glass spiked with crystal stars

honking horns
headlight beams
voices screaming
wailing sirens

cut away dress and lace
stretcher, first aid
screaming siren speed
Emergency Entrance

40 staples – titanium plate
narco-daze
whimper and moan
sweat and shiver

pulse
erratic
weak
precious

Poor poetry! A subject purposely avoided – Thanatophobia. Properly rejected by contest judges. A previous poem awarded Honorable Mention captures a scene where my darling wife caught dinner – two rainbow trout. Sad. No longer able to hike to Jade Lake. Fishing impossible! Sad. The destruction of life, reckless and foolish. The common curse, a highway infectious disease – D.U.I. – 100% preventable disease.

A Pretty Little Lake

a jade teardrop
cut into a granite mountain
reflecting corkscrew spires
dinosaurian boulders

clouds skip across, skirts flying
the morning sun smoldering

crimson blue smoke
reeds whistling a fairy cant

autumn leaves, fire-burst gold
orange fur-balls, twin bobcats
tempted by rainbows
green crystals searching pools
black logs slumbering on white sand
Sasquatch footprints cast in mud
red hawk watching from a tree top
patient, motionless, wary

impuissant sounds magnified by solitude
echoes bragging of eternity
a vast space filled with the clutter of time
a place spirits call home

survival of inhabitant
linked to happen-chance
directed by the Grand Master
too busy to reveal a face

February 3rd

Letter to our lawyer. D.d. court date scheduled February 10th. Please advise concerning court attendance and statement?

Picture the d.d, sipping beer, listening to counsel. The grown-up world. Play along. Neat, sincere, apology for mayhem – college bound. Prefers the dark brew, cold mug. A success story

Recent d.d. female, age twenty-one, wrong way direction on freeway. Six killed. A family, the sister and friend of the d.d. Convicted of d.d. at age seventeen.

D.d. teen court date, seven days. Justice!

February 4th
Angel baseball, promotional game. College challenge.

Knee injury, limited flexibility, pain day and night at rest.
Back continued pain, nerves aggravate stomach – digestion.
Shoulder therapy continues.

A chubby little roly-poly doll turned into a plastic Barbie that cries ouch when touched. No more beach walks, forest trails. Retirement woe! Never anticipate smooth sailing where rogue waves flow.

Angels won!

February 5th
Pain management therapy.
One night away – sick to stomach. Argument about length of future vacation plan – travel adjustment. A future forget-it-all, get-away recommended by our lawyer.
Insurance settlement and lawsuit – litigation continues.
D.d. trial postponed one, two, three times. Why?
Third prosecutor assigned. Why?

February 6th

A hammock moon. Clouds after a rain. No more camping. The tent tucked away. We have each other, each day. The kisses, hugs, laughter.

The d.d. switched us off the main track, we're on a spur. Slower pace, less landscape, marginal excitement. More ache and pain, less rock-and-roll.

Insurance increase liability and underinsured motorist. My car needs an air-bag. Old enough to figure, I've beat the odds on death. My dad died at fifty. Male ancestors died young in my family history. Average life expectance for my wife's ancestors – good.

Reality Play:

Play… Scene One… Crash with car showing an emergency rescue. Crash sounds.

Play… Scene Two… Phone message… Sad news. Death/ Injury?

Play… Scene Three. Police and three teens. D.U.I. caught. Walking the line.

Dialogue:

"6,000 crashes in the L.A. area in January and February. Down slightly from last year."

Movie:

Based on True Story

Hollywood child star, crossing the street, killed by D.U.I.

February 7th

Child actor, retired, killed in crosswalk by D.U.I. Headline morning newspaper.

Danger crossing a street in modern America.

Television showed a teen girl struck by two cars while in a crosswalk. Car hit-and-ran.

Trivialize crash scenes. The incredible violent destruction. Ants bumping heads on the road to yesterday.

Medical document sent to lawyer prove the physical harm. Damned pain. Tiredness!

Life is damaged recklessly.

Dreams transfer information on a cellular level. The toe feels the kick in the dream and the feeling exists in every cell. Pain in the back, ever cell an electric shock, over and over. Seven healthy survivors. My poor darling wounded by the grenade.

A new drunk in Texas chased by police – killed two people. No money for bail.

Ontology – branch of metaphysics studying existence.

February 8th

The diary evolved into dread, my darling wife ravaged by a d.d. Months of pain, pain, more pain. The human spirit becomes childlike. Prickly Bush, where Roses once grew. The unjust result of a dumb, blind mind.

The gift of life tips the scale toward grace and harmony. We have time to heal. Faith in God's kindness. The beauty of the stars. Our hearts, together.

February 9th

Tomorrow, the Criminal Trial to decide justice for the d.d. that slashed my wife on October 20th. And bashed her beautiful body brutally. Eight people escaped death.

I see the faces of the party drinkers – drunk – unconcerned by the misery they caused. No penalty? A freeway fender-bender in a Construction Zone. My wife survived a high speed collision into a concrete wall – twice!

Highway Headlines
People Insane in the Fast Lane

Who hit and killed the son of a judge?
$100,000 reward for information.

Two students in crosswalk struck by D.U.I.
Drunk driver records lost by police.

Zodiac Radio a.m. 5:30 – T.G.I.F.
Happy hour, devil brew, double!

February 10th – Criminal Trial
A cruel age, where compassion supercedes justice.

Radio: Traffic Clear
Crash cleared east on the 91
Clear drive on 605
Police arrest driver for D.U.I.
Ambulance siren – sharp and clear

Play Title – **A Bump in the Road – Road Kill – Chalk on the Sidewalk**

A child killed in a car chase. Twenty-six year old evading the police. Civil Rights of victim – highway safety – violated. Rigid laws, disciplined, straight. Uniform justice.

Verdict?

February 11th

Bus crash, ten died, five teens. Double trailer, cross the line.

Full moon. Pain dominates daily new reality. Doctor visits, medication, therapy, tears. Stomach disorder, weight loss, fear. Cold, cold, cold.

A new day with a new word for a new poem. Not anymore.

Help to lift my wife from bed – moans and groans. Massage to relax her back. Her apology for her weakness. Pain across the chest.

The number of D.U.I. crimes this year? One million?

"Pains are flinging her about like an old rag, a filthy torn rag doll" Vicki Baum

February 12th

Over the weekend, four teens killed by a d.d. on the freeway. Three in the morning leaving a party.

One teen killed in her bedroom by a d.d. crashing into her home, after midnight.

Back rub, ice pack, pain/inflammation medication. "I'm going to lay down." New mantra. A new direction, forced direction, the road of a D.U.I. victim.

Healthy, comfortable sex, now a single painful experience.

Four drunks on our highway racing away from the first collision. Dark, no witness, accelerate. One car blocking the escape route.

Two older ladies, early start on a vacation.

War injuries expatiates the death of our warriors. The highway battlefield is equally vicious on innocent victims of D.U.I. crimes. Domestic terror!

Approval for Pain Management Classes. God Bless my wife. She tries so hard but the pain continues.

February 13th

A year is a critical time for recovery of serious injury. Disruption of recovery process is avoided. Consistent, positive execution of daily performance. No surprises. A year, precious as the first year of a baby.

Controlled environmental condition.

Comfort zone – familiarity.

Proper nutrition.

Exercise.

Emotional stability.

Altercation of practiced, orderly procedures day and night is counter productive to recovery and maintenance of health.

Security of health care response is essential.

"Reason in man is rather like God in the world." St. Thomas Aquinas

February 14th – Valentine's Day
The slow retreat of daytime heat,
107, 106, 105…
The slow retreat of weight.
104, 103, 102…

Bless you Darling.
Please, be my Valentine.
Heart to Heart
A precious kiss

Deep, deep love
Tenderness
My Valentine

The personal fear and pain from injury shared by the brave.

A day of carnage on the highway, D.U.I. celebration. The holiday highway, deadly as a battlefield. Destructive as a tank blast.

Sad, sad, sad.

Extreme concern for weight loss. Physical deterioration frightening. A healthy, fleshy, vigorous woman destroyed. Slow, apathy, always tired in pain, skeletal.

My wife's frail face smiling. Her face is the angel.

Curse the face of her assassin, the devil.

Denture problems. The loss of weight affect on the body.

My Valentine!

Curling into a fetal ball. Fragile thread of life. Afraid to write another line. Are the negative thoughts projecting future conditions? God! The weight. Writing these words I'm crying. I'm miserable.

February 15th
Weight loss!

She is weak, tired. At night her breathing gentle as an Angle feather touching lips.

I touch her cold hand and pray.

We do not deserve punishment for the avoidable D.U.I. crime. And, does the villain escape justice?

Maturity does not reap wisdom. Anger and vengeance ripens with age. A curse on the d.d. Fool, asshole, fucker, bastard, dumb, damn d.d. creep. Words! Words don't kill like drunk drivers – the sons-of-bitches.

Anger is a deadly poison to the body. With each page written, anger weakens the spirit. Pages of pain; pages of anger. Confusion and ignorance guiding the pen. Justice questionable. Stop crying! *Fireman, age 25, killed by drunk driver.* Pray for the new victim.

February 16th
Knee surgery postponed. Weight gain essential to insure successful surgery.

Surgery resulting from the drunk driver collision, near death for eight humans. Medical and legal turmoil continuing. The consistent factor – pain!

Present condition fragile.

Pain and suffering because four drunks decide to cruise the freeway after a night of party drinking. A cocktail at sunrise for death. Pain! Fear and anger!

To relieve pain, back surgery recommended to repair fracture and chips on spine. After weight gain, after knee surgery.

The cold facts. Eight humans survive death. Relief to survive. On with life. One detour, the road of pain – my wife.

Too many lives damaged by the drunk driver.

D.U.I. crime is 100% preventable.

God Bless the Highway Victim.

February 17th
Three hours delay by pharmacist for pain drugs. Two trips in traffic to fill prescription. Pills take time to package

and deliver. Protections and precautions prevent misuse of drugs. Wait in line.

Alcohol is America's number one treatment for pain. Easy to obtain, no lines, no prescription. Extremely effective.

Letter to lawyer; decision on Civil Trial. Poem of collision sent to Writer's Digest Writing Competition. My wife did not proofread the poem. Transmission of thoughts of negative influence, recalling D.U.I. collision avoided.

Thanatophobia a problem.

Pain a problem.

Justice determined a problem.

February 18th – Future

Imagine the future nursing home. Recovery with nano robotics treatment to fix a problem. Cloned parts for replacement. Computer synthesizer controlling pain. Virtual reality exercise equipment – a bicycle ride along the beach. All inclusive diagnostic scanner, hand held ray – like on **Star Trek**.

Windows to see the sky. Wall panels, sterile. Air cleanser, purification. Water treatment facility. Pool, sauna, steam bath. Ice machine.

Imagine the rehab center for the Texas teen D.U.I. (10 years probation) – a mother and her daughter killed. Modern technology. Sauna. Golf course! Tennis!

The D.U.I. attend a MADD presentation. MADD mothers have nothing to celebrate. The highway D.U.I. terrorist is as vicious and destructive as yesterday.

Big business for courts. Premium bonus for insurance agencies.

Grief, loss, disbelief for the D.U.I. victim.

February 19th

"A life indifferent as a star." Randall Jarrell

Highway death, death so common, like disease and war, the reason obscure or senseless or patriotic. Death by D.U.I. a stupid death. D.U.I. death, the death lottery anyone can lose.

Winter days quick to dissolve. Winter is often short. The d.d. will laugh at his teenage foolery, never to acknowledge or regret the D.U.I. crime. Smoke!

Positive thought, make-up a happy future. Health! Fun! No Pain! Leave the graveyard of D.U.I. victims. Live!

Burn the diary. Burn the past. Start new.

February 20th, 21st, 22nd...

Waiting: knee surgery – back surgery...

Weight: 98 – 97 – 95...

Scream...

End Diary

********** ********** ********** **********

XIV

Final Statement

FINAL STATEMENT

The diary is a very personal recording, a personal warning to our family. A warning to the honest motorist, respecting the highway laws. Today a girl, age four, killed by a twenty-six year old drunk driver. So many innocent deaths. Passengers without the safety of an advanced model automobile suffer incredibly consequences in collisions – fragile hearts when flesh and metal collide. Thank God for air bag technology. My wife and her friend survived. The airbag did not save the small girl. The drunk driver failed to stop. Modern technology will stop cars automatically to avoid collision. The greatest technologic advance cannot replace respect for the law, respect for the rights of people, respect for life.

Was justice served for inflicting a violent collision driving drunk? The legal system cannot deter D.U.I. crime with a policy of leniency. Acceptance of limited punishment for the D.U.I. criminal is compassionate. The liquor advertisement posted behind home plate during the World Series defines the

American position on alcohol and youth. Insurance lawyers defending the drunk driver, without defense of the passenger victim is unfair, especially considering the source of the defense fund – deducted from honest motorist's insurance payments.

Our lawyer apologized to us for the D.U.I. verdict.

"I apologize for our legal system and its many complexities. There have been considerable changes to the legal system over my forty years of practice, some for the good and some for the bad. But, it is our system, and it is still the best in the world. Thank you. Very truly yours, (lawyer name)."

Tuesday – A news flash, car crash into a home, killing a child – six – asleep in bed. 22 year old female D.U.I. Her statement of defensive driving to avoid vehicle collision with an erratic driver. Loss of control – crash through wall of house.

Violent death, years of news and movie violence, awful, awful, awful. Powerless reaction. D.U.I. is a bother, justice will be lenient.

This week, three dead in D.U.I. collisions. Three children: age one, three, six. Innocent voices silenced. Lifelines extinguished. Every week a day of D.U.I. death.

Drink responsibly? Perhaps advertise an adult product responsibly. Booze for sale behind home plate in the World Series is greed! Damn the bastards! And damn the teams promoting alcohol while a number one super star player is at bat. No wins! The curse? What can be done! The curse of the MADD Witch!

Wednesday – Nineteen year old female killed by drunk driver in Riverside.

Thursday – Pro football player arrested for D.U.I. Released on his own recognizances.

Friday – Policeman assisting trucker struck by D.U.I. on 91-Freeway.

Saturday – Drunk driver kills man at bus stop. Four previous D.U.I. convictions.

Sunday – Top golf professional arrested for D.U.I. Refused to take breathalyzer test.
Released on own recognizances. Celebrity rehab. Press blackout. No pain.

Monday – Grandfather killed in bedroom by nineteen year old D.U.I. driver of van.

People maimed, futures ruined, pain. A twice convicted D.U.I. criminal celebrity receives a good citizen award. Justice, common sense superseded by greed – sponsors selling whiskey, wine and beer.

Three days, three weeks, three months. Time for recovering, time for healing, time for suffering. Weakness and pain. Present fear – weight loss! If weight were money, my wife is bankrupt. Weight loss scary. Shuffle walk; weak smile. Sad words, "pain is depressing me."

The number of lives wrecked by the D.U.I. criminal daily increases. A trail of grief and suffering – 100% preventable.

The D.U.I. criminal justice is lenient. Forgive the fool that drank too much. Who hasn't? Accept the carnage and murder. Premeditated choice to roll the dice of death. 2000 pounds of steel projectile filled with high octane fuel.

The drunk driver gets a free ride, starting with the pat on the head to prevent a bump entering the police vehicle. Bail by friends or relatives. Counsel by insurance lawyers. Defended by the public defender; prosecuted by the public prosecutor. Minimal jail time, minimal fine. Free to return to drink and drive. Probation. Expensive process, our tax money spent wisely.

We pray for the highway victims. We pray for a future without D.U.I. pain. God Bless the Highway Victims.

Final words for the Miracle Workers. Heroes struggling to save a life stricken on an American highway. God bless the police, emergency and medical workers. God bless you! God bless you! God bless you!

Respectfully,

The Highway Victim

*********** *********** *********** *********

XV

Fourth Letter to Our Lawyer

Dear Lawyer:

Responding to your request for physical copy of medical costs.

Catered Manor bill: $17,892.15
UCI bill: $187,107.00
Surgeon bill: $8,104.00
Continuing medical treatment costs not included. Knee surgery/back surgery pending
Out of pocket cost for shower chair, hospital bed rental, donut cushion, travel cost, medication, knee brace, hot patches, ice packs – money deducted from retirement savings.

Therapy continues. The surgeon said the therapy will hurt. Pain continues. Reevaluation next month. Appearance is deceptive. Internal complication, invisible injury. Bone chips and fractures. Movement without pain is impossible. No sleeping on left side. Her knee in pain Back aching. All symptoms undetectable by the eye.

Regarding recent conference concerning Civil Trial. Thank you for the information. Our decision to continue Civil Trial for the drunk driver is inconclusive at this time. Continued medical treatment is exhausting. Knee surgery and back surgery scheduling problem – weight concern by surgeons.

The insurance agencies commitment to defend the rights of the drunk driver is discouraging. Public acceptance of the D.U.I. tragedies makes a jury selection for the injury victim a challenge. The question of reasonable restitution for pain and suffering is difficult to determine. Is a professional soccer player's arm expendable? Will the beer logo on the back of his shirt adversely influence the jury?

Good news for the drinking motorist. No loss of license to drive. No loss of driving insurance. No jail time. No restrictions on alcohol consumption. Free criminal defense by Public Defender. Free Civil Defense by an Automobile Insurance Agency like Progress, Multi-State and Infinite. No loss of job – discrimination. On parole? No worry – no return to jail for D.U.I. criminality – guarantee! All good news. The bar is open!

Blame for failure to stop the D.U.I. calamity is distributed between major societal constructs: medical, legal, liquor industry, insurance, advertisement, college, culinary trade, legal, political. And motorist apathy and sympathy for son and daughter, neighbor and friend – the drinking crowd – is commendable but ineffective deterring the D.U.I.

Lack of response to help stop the D.U.I. on American highways is unconsciousable by the individual. The groups divide the blame with conviction of reason. And, convince the honest motorist to accept the D.U.I. condition on American highways without possibility of total prevention. Effort to prevent D.U.I. limited to MADD and the occasional public warning. Have you ever seen an insurance agency advertisement directed at the D.U.I. tragedy? Check your insurance policy, not a word about D.U.I. danger on the highway.

Commitment by the public to ban cigarette advertising should extend to alcohol. No cigarettes on the comic page. Alcohol impacts millions of lives negatively. Vandalism, abuse, drunk driving, fights, suicide – alcohol influence evident. The World Series advertisement banner behind home plate – major beer brand in bold red letters and a bold logo like a baseball decal. Impressive! Next inning sign shifts to auto insurance. Nasty hypocrite!

The legal procedure for Civil Court is complex with multiple obstacles to deter the conviction of a drunk driver. Medical records are not proof of injury. X-ray of injury might be faked. A doctor must testify at considerable cost. Doctors never donate time to testify in a D.U.I. Civil Trail. All medical testimony paid by injury victim is challenged by medical experts provided by drunk driver's insurance provider.

The Civil Trial forbids identification of D.U.I. criminality since the Progress lawyer directed the drunk driver to accept liability for injury. It is understandable policy. The jury would probably be unfairly influenced to discover my wife's injuries resulted from a collision caused by a teen drunk driver in a Construction Zone – minimal insurance despite lack of driving experience and a reckless driving charge.

The identity of the Insurance Agency providing the lawyer for the drunk driver is forbidden to be revealed to the jury. Understandable! This diary cannot be read by a jury. Understandable!

Winning the Civil Claim will result in immediate bankruptcy by the teen drunk driver. Poverty is the best insurance. Also, a percentage of medical cost is deducted from settlement funds. My wife contributed to her medical insurance during her years of work for L.A. County. The drunk teen driver never worked.

The Civil Trial like the Criminal Trial does nothing to combat D.U.I. collisions on American Highways. In fact, the legal system protects the rights of the drunk driver. In most collisions the victim with the neck injury is probably lying to gain insurance money. Limited Progress policy is valid as legal restitution to injured passenger struck by Progress insured teenage drunk driver.

The criminal act of D.U.I. is equal to Rape and Murder. The D.U.I. victim traumatized in a death spiral, severe and shocking memory branded in the brain. The body condemned to permanent torture. A regiment of drugs to maintain pain control and balance a fragile health.

The three insurance agencies refuse reasonable settlement for victims and defend the convicted drunk driver policy as the Gold Standard for D.U.I. Request for D.U.I. Policy Statement (Mission Statement), the request was ignored.

Millions of dollars collected from drunk driver policies reinstating the convicted D.U.I. motorist at a premium cost; no additional coverage required to protect honest motorists of repeat D.U.I. collision.

A lawsuit to challenge the inadequate teen coverage provided by insurance agencies is impossible. Minimum coverage for convicted D.U.I. motorists is acceptable insurance policy. Insurances agencies have unlimited funds for legal cost to defend d.d. policy. Request for reasonable restitution challenged by legal experts. A trial decision for the victim, expect appeal?

Obviously, failure to provide insurance against the D.U.I. is the responsibility of the motorist. There is no national law to protect the passenger victim of D.U.I. In fact, the laws exhibit compassion and leniency for the drunk driver. A drunk driver shares the same highway privilege as a trucker of cab driver – insurance identical. Underinsured or uninsured acceptable policy to defend drunk criminal drivers.

The jury will never read the diary. The jury will never read the names of the people that saved a life. The cause of the pain irrelevant. The jury will never reflect on the courage of the victim, the pain. Each day the message is repeated, pain. And, the pain is the same today as in the beginning. The weight loss is killing her and killing me. D.U.I. tragedy is repeated across our nation.

The d.d. is driving, highway privilege restored. Repair of damaged D.U.I. car, supplied by insurance coverage by Progress. Capable of insurance cost; a free man. Bankruptcy follows the Civil Trial. Two years of bad credit the d.d.

penalty. Settlement cost – zero. Cost of Civil Trial defense provided by Progress insurance expert lawyers. Cost to D.U.I. – zero.

Our cost to provide the doctor to testify is thousands of dollars. Our cost for legal representations is thousands of dollars. Tough choice? The Civil Trial, a recording of justice with no justice served.

Discouraging information. Continued legal costs are considerable. Civil Trial costly. We are committed to receive justice for the horrific collision by the drunk driver. After knee surgery and back surgery medical costs assessed, continued legal action will be determined.

Thank you for the information. Our final decision for Civil Trial pending knee surgery and back surgery result.

God Bless the Highway Victims.

Respectfully,

The Highway Victim

********** ********** ********** **********

XVI

D.U.I. Criminal Verdict & Sentence

JUDGEMENT

Orange County
OC Probation

(Name)
Chief Probation Officer
Telephone (714) 000-0000

909 N. Main St.
Santa Ana, CA

Mailing Address
P.O Box 10260
Santa Ana, CA 92711-0260

Date: XX/00/0000

Defendant: Xxxx
C-111000
Court No. 11FG0000

Court Date: XX/00/0000
Incident Date: October 20/0000

Dear Ms. Victim:

Post Disposition Letter

The Orange County Probation Department previously requested a victim impact statement from you or a member of your family prior to the above-named defendant's sentencing hearing. The investigating Deputy Probation Officer may have sent a "Notice of Sentencing Proceedings" letter and, in some cases, made a follow-up telephone call. This letter follows any previous contacts. This letter notifies you of the defendant's sentence in this case and summarizes any rights you may have to restitution.

On XX/00/0000, the Superior Court of Orange County conducted a sentencing hearing involving the defendant. The checked mark below shows the disposition of the defendant's case.

Case Findings

X "No legal cause why judgment should not be pronounced and defendant having Pled Guilty to Count 1. Imposition of sentence is suspended and defendant is placed on three year(s) FORMAL PROBATION on the following terms and conditions.

X *Serve 180 Day(s) Orange County Jail as to Count 1.

X Complete 95 Day(s) Caltrans/Physical Labor in lieu of 180 days jail as directed by Probation Department Defendant to complete 95 days as follows. 50 days Caltrans/physical labor and 45 days community service for a total of 95 days, as to Counts 1.

X Pay restitution in the amount as determined and directed by Probation Department as to Count 1. Court orders all monies paid applied to restitution first.

* Please contact the Orange County Probation Department regarding the name of the defendant's assigned probation officer.

* Please refer to attached VICTIM WITNESS pamphlet for more information. (Only applies to case involving victims of violence.)

As a victim or victim's next of kin, you are entitled to review the sentencing recommendations in the probation report. If you decide to review the sentencing recommendation, please contact the Victim Witness Assistance Program in the Court where the case was heard.

If the defendant is sentenced to state prison and you would like to receive notification regarding the parole hearing date or proposed release date from the California Department of Corrections and Rehabilitation (CDC&R), please contact the CDC&R directly by mailing a completed form CDCR 1707. The form is available on-line at http:///www.cdcr. ca.gov/Victim Services/application html, or the form may be obtained from any Victim Witness Program office.

If the defendant is sentenced to the Orange County jail and you would like information on the proposed release date, please telephone the VINE (Victim Information and Notification Everyday} hotline at l-800-721-8021.

For your information, in accordance with the laws of this state, a person who is sentenced to time in custody is entitled to "conduct or work time credits." These credits can reduce by one-third is one-half the actual amount of time a person spends in custody on the sentence imposed by the Court.

In addition to the above rights, you may be entitled to restitution for your losses. Restitution may be collected from the defendant who committed the crime against you or made available to you from the state restitution fund.

* If the Court place the defendant on supervised probation (formal), the Orange County Probation Department will attempt to collect restitution on your behalf.

* If the Court place the defendant on unsupervised probation (informal), the Victim Witness Assistance Program will attempt to collect restitution on your behalf.

* If the defendant was sentenced to State Prison, and the Court ordered restitution at the time of sentencing, restitution may be collected through the California Department of Corrections.

California Department of Corrections
Office of Victim Services and Restitution

P.O. Box 942883
Sacramento, CA 94283-0001
Phone: (916) 358-2436 or Toll Free: (877) 256-6877

* The Victims of Crime Program is the "payer of last resort." The primary source revenue for the program is derived from the imposition and collection of restitution fines and penalty assessments levied against convicted offenders. To contact the Victims of Crime Program, please call toll free (800) 777-9229.

If you have any further questions regarding the defendant sentence or the information contained in this letter, please contact (name), Supervising Probation Officer.

Very truly yours,

(Name)
Deputy Probation Officer 00000
1 (714) 000-0000
FAX: 1 (714) 000-0000

********** ********** **********

Case Summary

Case Number:	111FG0000
OC Pay Number:	0000000
Originating Court:	North
Defendant:	Xxxx,
Demographics:	

Eyes:	Brown
Hair:	Black
Height:	5' 9"
Weight (lb)	152

Names

Last Name	First Name	Middle Name	Type
Xxxx	Xxxx	Xxxx	Real Name

Case Status:

Status:	Convicted
Case Stage:	
Release Status:	Released on Bail
Warrant:	N
DMV Hold:	N
Charging Document:	Complaint
Mandatory Appearance:	Y
Owner's Resp:	N
Amendment #:	1

Counts:

Seq	S/A	Violation Date	Section Statute	OL	Violation	Plea
1)		XX/00/0000	23153(a)	VCF	Driving under influence alcohol/drug with injury	Guilty
1	1	XX/00/0000	12022.7(a)	PCF	ENH-Inflict Great Bodily Harm	Admitted

Plea Date	Disposition	Disposition Date
XX/00/0000	Pled Guilty	XX/00/0000
XX/00/0000	Admission	XX/00/0000

Participants:

Role	Badge Agency	Name
District Attorney	OCDA	(Name)
Retained Attorney	RETAT	(Name),
District Attorney	OCDA	(Name)
District Attorney	OCDA	(Name)
District Attorney	OCDA	(Name)

DUI Case – Judgement Verdict

Public Defender	OCPD	(Name)
District Attorney	OCDA	(Name)

Heard Hearings:

Date Hearing Type – Reason Courtroom Hearing Status: Special Hearing Result

XX/00/0000 Arraignment in Custody	C11 Heard	
XX/00/0000 Pre Trial	N12 Heard 10 court/60 calendar days	
XX/00/0000 Preliminary Hearing	N12 Cancel	
XX/00/0000 Pre Trial Disposition & Reset	N12 Heard Reasonable Time Waiver	
XX/00/0000 Preliminary Hearing	N12 Cancel	
XX/00/0000 Pre Trial Disposition & Reset	N12 Heard Reasonable Time Waiver	
XX/00/0000 Pre Trial Disposition & Reset	N12 Heard Reasonable Time Waiver	
XX/00/0000 Pre Trial Disposition & Reset	N12 Heard	
XX/00/0000 Pre Trial Disposition & Reset	N12 Heard	

Bail:

Bail Date Post Amount Available Amount Depositor Depositor Address Details

	Action	Action Date	Amount
	Active	XX/00/0000	50000
	Exonerated	XX/00/0000	0
XX/00/0000 50000 (Name)	Reopened	XX/00/0000	0
	Applied	XX/00/0000	1600
	Exonerated	XX/00/0000	0

Sentences:

Seq # Sentence Date Sentence

1　XX/00/0000　3 years Probation

2　XX/00/0000　*180 days jail

3　XX/00/0000　95 days Service in lieu of jail

4　XX/00/0000　$390.00 Fines

5　XX/00/0000　Restitution

6　XX/00/0000　3 months First Offender Alcohol Program

7　XX/00/0000　Youthful Drug and Alcohol Deterrence

8　XX/00/0000　Mothers Against Drunk Driving (MADD) Victim's Impact Panel

Probation:

Sent Seq #	Type	Term	End Date
1	Formal	3 years	XX/00/0000

History:

Status	Status Date	End Date
Active	XX/00/0000	XX/00/0000

********** ********** ********** **********

XVII

D.U.I. Crime is 100% Preventable

VICTIM'S JUSTICE – Propositions to Prevent D.U.I. Crime.

1... Sobriety Law. Three Day Incarceration from time of arrest. Incarceration during withdrawal and hangover symptoms – dizziness, headache, lack of muscle control, sleepy – alcohol incapacitation resulting in danger to public safety. Three day jail watch before bail. Jail costs from insurance coverage.

2... D.U.I. Criminal Identification Logo on Car License Plate and Driver License. Clear I.D. Logo like the Handicap Sticker – Wheelchair on victim's license plates.

3... Court Judgement! No Alcohol Consumption. Restricted Alcohol Consumption. Legal control of Alcoholic Consumption. Mandatory attendance of A.A.

4... Mandatory increase in convicted D.U.I. driver's Auto Coverage to protect honest motorists. Provide reasonable restitution for D.U.I. victims by the Insurance Industry. Poor and wealthy motorists receive equal protection against the D.U.I. tragedy on American Highways. Pedestrian and passenger coverage, financed by D.U.I. insurance premium.

5... Passenger accountability when traveling with a drunk driver. Restricted license. Insurance notification. Fine. Driver class – MADD.

6... Internet identification site for criminal D.U.I. like the sex offender site. Specify driving routes and car identity. No personal information.

7... Restriction of alcohol advertisement impressed on youth and children. No beer banner behind home plate in the World Series. No beer plug during a Super Bowl champion's appreciation speech. Professional soccer player's beer name on shirts – out. Cigarette restriction in advertisement is an effective model.

8... Minimum of five year probation for first offense of D.U.I. crime. Jail term determined by victims of D.U.I. crime.

9... All medical cost of injury and burial cost paid by drunk driver and D.U.I. insurance

10... Mission Statement to address the elimination of D.U.I. crime by responsible leaders – culinary, sports, advertisement, liquor, insurance, political, legal, medical, college and public.

11... Warning on liquor labels. *Excessive alcohol consumption may cause irrational, abusive and violent behavior. Addictive!* D.U.I. warning signs where liquor sold.

12... 20 hours of driving training; test with D.M.V. before driving privilege restored.

********** ********** ********** **********

God Bless the Highway Victims

If Everyone

If everyone who drive a car
Could lie a month in bed,
With broken bones and stitched-up wounds,
Or fractures of the head.
And there endure the agonies
That many people do.
They'd never need preach safety
Anymore to me or you.

If everyone could stand beside
The bed of some close friend
And hear the Doctor say "No Hope"
Before that fatal end,
And see him there unconscious
Never knowing what took place,
The laws and rules of traffic
I am sure we'd soon embrace.

If everyone could meet
The wife and children left behind
And step into the darkened home
Where once the sunlight shined,
And look upon "the Vacant Chair,"
Where Daddy used to sit,
I am sure each reckless driver
Would be forced to think a bit.

If everyone who takes the wheel
Would say a little prayer,
And keep in mind those in the car
Depending on his care,
And make a vow and pledge himself
To never take a chance,
The Great Crusade for Safety
Would suddenly advance.

Author unknown

Printed in the United States
By Bookmasters